A Prescription for Wellness:

Health Behaviors That Improve Outcomes after Breast Cancer

New Life *after* Cancer

Author

New Life *after* Cancer

A 501c3 non-profit charitable organization, our goal is to teach and support health practices that have been proven to improve outcomes after breast cancer through small-group retreats, workshops, and lectures.

Instructors

Carolyn I. Sartor, MD
Elizabeth Janks, LMSW, ACSW
Doreen Stein-Seroussi, MA, MPH, RYT
Angela Diebolt, BFA
Loretta Muss, RN
Laura Gasaway, MLS, JD
Valerie Collins, PT, CLT-LANA

Who We Are

Cancer Survivors
Oncologists
Academicians
Community Practitioners
Friends and Family of Survivors

ISBN-10: 153714555X
ISBN-13: 978-1537145556

About the Contributors

Carolyn I. Sartor, MD is past Professor and Chair of the Department of Radiation Oncology at the University of North Carolina School of Medicine, and co-Director of the Breast Cancer Program at UNC/Lineberger Comprehensive Cancer Center. A translational scientist, she designed and implemented clinical trials stemming from her laboratory research discoveries. As a nationally recognized leader, she has served on the executive boards of committees directing breast cancer clinical trials, education, and research, including Cancer and Leukemia Group B (CALGB), American Society of Therapeutic Radiation Oncology (ASTRO), and American Association for Cancer Research (AACR). She has given cancer center Grand Round and Visiting Professor lectures at many prestigious universities, nationally and internationally. She has published extensively in medical literature, and contributed to the textbooks "Breast Cancer: A Guide to Fellows" and "Clinical Radiation Oncology". She is a breast cancer survivor.

Elizabeth Janks, LMSW, ACSW is the Associate Director of Training for MI-DDI at Wayne State University. She holds a Master's degree in social work with both national and state certification. Her specialty is in helping people to identify person-directed action plans that facilitate meaningful life changes. Through supporting her niece and sister-in-law's breast cancer journeys, she decided to adapt her expertise to breast cancer survivorship. She has taught at the New Life *after* Cancer What Now retreats.

Angela Diebolt, BFA graduated from the University of Michigan School of Fine Arts. In New Life *after* Cancer retreats she develops creative tools for self-awareness.

Doreen Stein-Seroussi, MA, MPH, RYT is the lead yoga instructor at the UNC/Lineberger Comprehensive Cancer Center's Cancer Survivorship Program. She received her initial Kripalu-based yoga training and certification in 2003, is a Yoga Alliance Registered Yoga Teacher, and a member of the International Association of Yoga Therapists. Doreen teaches yoga for cancer survivors and their families at Cornucopia Cancer Support Center and at UNC Cancer Support Program. She teaches gentle yoga classes and provides private yoga therapy for Duke Integrative Medicine. She has taught at the New Life *after* Cancer What Now retreats.

Loretta Muss, RN is the Coordinator of the Patient and Family Advisory Board for the North Carolina Cancer Hospital. Her passion for cooking led her to teach New Life *after* Cancer cooking classes, emphasizing the joy of cooking simple but healthy and delicious meals.

Laura Gasaway, MLS, JD is past Director of the University of North Carolina Law Library, Associate Dean of the School of Law, and a Professor of Law. Her professional expertise is in copyright law and library management. A breast cancer survivor, New Life *after* Cancer's programs changed her life. She has taught at the New Life *after* Cancer What Now retreats.

Valerie Collins, PT, CLT-LANA is a stout advocate of exercise for breast cancer survivors. As a physical therapist, she was one of the founding members of New Life *after* Cancer, leading the Arm against Lymphedema workshops. She is a certified lymphedema therapist for UNC Healthcare, specializing in breast cancer survivors.

Illustrators

Cover Artwork by **Beth Palmer.** Beth is active in both the arts education and arts in healthcare fields, and through her artwork is creating a new imaginative space where those areas connect. Her art and her life as an artist bring fresh perspective and openness to how we see our health, our lives and our relationships. After experiencing a cancer diagnosis and challenging side effects of treatments, Beth drew on her career as an art teacher to begin creating artwork that has been described as "joyful and colorful", "beautiful and provocative," and "insider-outsider art."

Sunshine was painted on a repurposed canvas. Beth applied cheese cloth over the rather bumpy old canvas to disguise it, but soon realized it reminded her of surgical gauze, and also noticed that the loosely woven fibers of the cheese cloth could represent how we are all woven together into one fabric. The yellow sun is from her collection of old crocheted doilies. The pink flowers are cut from one of the hand painted cotton scarves Beth designed for women with hair loss. The stems are made from samples of painted paper from her time teaching elementary art. The flowers are leaning toward each other, toward the sunshine, which depicts how we can all help one another. Beth applied gold leaf to the old wooden frame, like a warm hug around the painting.

Illustrations by **Allison Diebolt**, a 10th grade student who has been an artist for as long as she can remember. She has a passion for helping others and hopes her art someday can make an effect on the world.

Dedication

For all of the wonderful women we have met through
New Life *after* Cancer's workshops and retreats.
You are the inspiration behind this book.

Table of Contents

Preface

"What now, Doctor? Is there something that I should do to help keep my breast cancer from coming back?" Patients ask their oncologists these words of concern and hope upon completing treatment. Yet, even with years of training, experts often miss the opportunity to direct their patients to lifestyle changes that could indeed benefit their long-term health care.

In *A Prescription for Wellness*, authored by a dream team of six specialists, aims to answer patients' calling to proactively direct their daily health care. Leading the group is Dr. Sartor, who has the unique perspective of seeing cancer from both sides, as a physician and patient. Dr. Sartor, a Professor of Radiation Oncology specializing in breast cancer treatment, is also a scientist at the forefront of breast cancer research and treatment, has lead large clinical trials in breast cancer. She also lives the patient side of her own specialty, having an aggressive breast cancer that has been treated with surgery, chemotherapy and radiation therapy.

Her coauthors lend tremendous insight and verification to the lifestyle changes that can make a difference in long-term survival. Among them are D. Stein-Seroussi, a lead Yoga instructor, E. Janks, a Social Worker, L. Muss, a Nurse with a passion for cooking, L. Gasaway, an Associate Law School Dean and breast cancer survivor, and V. Collins, a Physical therapist and certified lymphedema therapist.

A Prescription for Wellness separates itself from other cancer and lifestyle books in that it speaks to both breast cancer survivors and health care professionals. To both audiences, the authors discuss applicable clinical data from medical literature, offering substantial validity to often overlooked holistic daily interventions.

"I should be dead by now", writes Dr. Sartor, "I had never realized how effective lifestyle factors can be!" The content of this unique book is not just advice and recommendations, it is a life lived experience for each of the authors, who now want to share their knowledge with all breast cancer patients.

Divided into five sections, A Prescription for Wellness is easy to understand with suggestions that are both practical and most importantly, attainable. The data-based guidelines demonstrate the correlation between lowering the recurrence of breast cancer and five important factors; weight, exercise, diet quality, yoga, and mindfulness-based stress reduction.

One of the most beneficial attributes of the authors' clearly defined wellness elements is that this lifestyle makes sense for any person striving for healthy living, and thus can be incorporated into any family's daily living, facilitating support, a "buddy-system" and higher compliance for the breast cancer survivor.

Because each factor is supported with scientific evidence from the medical literature, healthcare providers can offer their patients this lifestyle plan with confidence and conviction, as a way to improve post-breast cancer outcomes. Simultaneously, breast cancer survivors are guided, "to accept that which we cannot change and to change thoughts and habits that do not serve us well". This book, *A Prescription for Wellness,* is a must have reference for both health care providers and cancer survivors.

Alphonse Taghian, MD, PhD
Professor of Radiation Oncology, Harvard Medical School
Breast Service, Department of Radiation Oncology
Director, Lymphedema Research Program
Massachusetts General Hospital

Acknowledgements

It takes a village . . .

There are many people who have contributed to this work, which is the culmination of many New Life *after* Cancer workshops and retreats. To name just a few:

Thank you to Hana Johnson for her crucial assistance in turning a manuscript into a book, and to Eric Johnson for ushering ideas through Photoshop reality.

Thank you to participants of New Life *after* Cancer programs who have shared their stories.

Thank you to the Board of New Life *after* Cancer for guiding the process from beginning to end.

Thank you to the faculty of workshops and retreats, for volunteering your time and expertise to teach all of us.

Thank you to UNC/Lineberger Comprehensive Cancer Center and the V Foundation for start-up funds to launch New Life *after* Cancer.

Especially, thank you to those who have donated funds to allow us to bring this work to press.

Introduction

A teachable moment

Studies show that breast cancer survivors are hungry for information about things that **they** can do to help prevent breast cancer recurrence and improve quality of life after breast cancer treatment. The time after breast cancer treatment is deemed a "teachable moment" by behavioral scientists for making meaningful strides in improving lifestyles. In other words, the time after breast cancer diagnosis and treatment is a time when one is more apt to seek out information regarding things that one can do for health and wellness. It is also a time when one is highly likely to make good on intentions to change lifestyles and adopt healthier ways of living. We will show data that proves that breast cancer survivors can successfully undertake exercise regimens, dietary change, and stress reduction practices to a degree that is unusually high in health behavior studies. Breast cancer survivors are very motivated to adopt health behaviors that will improve outcomes.

Although studies have shown how effective behavioral education can be during this "teachable moment" after breast cancer, sadly, studies also show that far too few breast cancer survivors are getting the information that they want and need. A surprisingly small minority of breast cancer survivors are given health behavior recommendations after treatment. This means that although breast cancer survivors are open-minded to being given information, and that they are unusually likely to act on that information, this "teachable moment" is often missed.

What are the most effective practices that breast cancer survivors can adopt to improve outcomes after treatment? After treatment is completed, the majority of breast cancer survivors turn to the internet, mass media, or word of mouth to meet their information needs. There is a virtual avalanche of information out there. While there is a great deal of beneficial information available online, much that is untested, unproven, or even wrong. Separating out the wheat from the chaff is critical, and is an enormous task. When trying to follow every fad that comes along, it is impossible to focus on the few that are proven to make a difference.

Our approach is to go directly to the source material, the peer-reviewed medical literature, to validate what is presented, and also to cull the field to find those health behaviors that are currently shown to be most effective and relevant. It is imperative that the information given during this "teachable moment" is valid. Clear, concise instructions from an authoritative source are needed.

Certainly, there are many breast cancer books available to breast cancer survivors. While most of them do give clear and concise recommendations, the actual data behind those recommendations are rarely presented. Changing health behaviors is very hard. Change requires motivation. **Information motivates. Recommendations do not.**

Therefore, it is crucial to convey that there are well-performed clinical trials showing that lifestyle behaviors result in significant improvements in breast cancer outcomes. Epidemiologic studies demonstrate that avoiding weight gain after treatment results in significantly reduced risk of dying from breast cancer or other causes. A modest amount of exercise significantly reduces the relative risk of breast cancer death, and is associated with absolute survival benefits on the order of 6%. Eating well has been proven to be associated with similar significant survival benefits. Randomized controlled trials prove that yoga and mindfulness-based stress reduction result in significant improvements in quality-of-life and a wide range of psychological benefits.

Who needs to read this book?

Breast cancer survivors:

Perhaps you are a breast cancer survivor who has just made it through a grueling course of diagnosis, decision-making, surgery, chemotherapy, and radiation therapy. You have invested so much blood, sweat, and tears, and now it's over. Congratulations on a job well done!

Along with this not-so-pleasant journey of breast cancer treatment, perhaps you've come to the realization that there is still more that can be done. That returning to your pre-cancer way of life isn't necessarily the best thing to do. Maybe you should, would, and could live more health-fully, more consciously, so that you can both help your body to recover and also avoid lifestyle habits that may be putting you at greater risk of recurrence.

What do you do? Is it time to start a new diet or invest in shark cartilage? There is so much information out there, it can be overwhelming. This book will be your guide to specific recommendations that have been proven to improve outcomes after breast cancer treatment.

Health care providers:

Perhaps you are a physician who has dedicated your career to curing breast cancer. You have just helped your patient to make it through a long course of the most state-of the-art, advanced treatment. She sits on the examination table now as you congratulate her on her last day of radiation therapy. She looks at you with both relief and a twinge of fear as she says, "What now, doctor? Is there something that I should do help to keep my breast cancer from coming back?"

What do you say? The standard answer is, "Now we just watch and wait. If it doesn't come back in 5 or 10 years, we will know that you are cured." You will likely launch into a discussion about the follow up mammogram and physical exam schedule. You may even get into the rationale for not doing more aggressive surveillance such as screening CT scans or following tumor markers.

However, it's unlikely that you will give your patient a prescription for lifestyle behaviors that she can practice that have been shown in robust clinical trials to improve outcomes. Why? Because they didn't teach you this in medical school, residency, or in the many continuing education conferences you've attended since.

The goal of this book is to provide a complete and concise guide to medical literature pertaining to health behaviors after breast cancer treatment so that you can write that prescription for wellness on your patient's last day of treatment, and offer her a book to back it up.

How to use this book

This book was written while wearing two hats. One is the professorial cap and gown, the other is the sunhat and prosthetic bra. This book is designed to meet the needs of both breast cancer survivors and health professionals. Thus, we have attempted to create a "book within a book". In reality, there is a fair amount of overlap between the two, because our experience teaching New Life *after* Cancer programs leads us to conclude that breast cancer survivors are very sophisticated learners, regardless of educational background. Therefore, the discussion of the clinical data from medical literature is presented at a level for both the health care professional and the information-seeking breast cancer survivor. Introductory and in-depth discussions are presented in lay terms with more explanatory background information for those who are less familiar with some of the medically-related concepts.

For health care providers, the good news is that there is a succinct body of literature related to health behaviors and breast cancer outcomes. Mastering the current knowledge base is readily doable. In order to present the information in an easily accessible format for busy professionals, we have reviewed the several hundred articles in medical journals in order to present the data for the primary studies in specific "key study" sections. Key study sections allow health care professionals to readily reference the discussion of the most relevant medical literature. Concise summaries are offered for those who may wish to skip right to the final conclusions. Full references are provided for those who wish to review in detail the specific studies. We encourage the serious student to do so, specifically with an eye to new studies that are being published even as we write. The sections culminate in a prescription intended to be written by the health care provider and given to the patient at the time of completion of treatment, a prescription for their wellness.

For breast cancer survivors, this book is not intended as a quick-read, but as a guide to lifestyle changes. There is a great deal of information in this book, knowledge that we have been gathering over many years. We suggest that you take it in slowly, bit by bit. As with many health initiatives, if you build up slowly, you accomplish far more meaningful change. To reinforce the gradual assimilation of new health behaviors as you progress, each part includes a self-assessment so that you can gauge your starting point. Each part also sets out specific recommendations as calls to action. Tracking your progress over time can be extremely valuable. Something as straightforward as writing down how many servings of vegetables you eat each day can have a significant influence on increasing your vegetable intake, and eating more healthfully overall. We suggest that you add each new call to action while continuing the ones you have already started. They are intended to build upon each other. If you digest the information gradually, while implementing new practices, you will be amazed at how lasting and far reaching the changes will be.

Breast cancer is a strong motivator

Changing behaviors is hard. If you've ever tried to quit smoking (good for you!), tried to diet, tried to exercise regularly, you know what we mean. Have you ever started a new lifestyle practice only to find that you keep it up for a short time and then lapse? Maybe you're motivated at first, but then the motivation fades. Maybe you're overwhelmed by the choices, doing first this, then that, getting slightly manic as the barrage of daily subscription emails toss you first one way then the next. Maybe you have good intentions at the outset, but the daily grind of sticking to a difficult routine wears you down. Maybe it's a matter of boredom, of not being able to or wanting to sustain the routine once it is no longer new or novel. Like the rest of us, you've probably tried to change your health behaviors in the past and failed. We reiterate: changing behaviors is hard. Fortunately, there are some compelling reasons why you **can** make significant health behavior changes this time.

In the past, you may have tried to lose those extra pounds in order to look better, or, feel better. That's a laudable goal, and reasonably motivating. But what if you've had breast cancer, just gone through extensive treatment, and you are told that changing your lifestyle can significantly improve breast cancer outcomes, reduce your risk of breast cancer recurrence, and even significantly improve survival? In other words, you're keeping those pounds off to **live!** That's what we call motivation. Breast cancer is a strong motivator to change.

We will show data that proves that breast cancer survivors can adhere to even the most stringent diets, when it is rare to see such compliance. Breast cancer survivors are very motivated to adopt health behaviors that will improve outcomes.

Keep it simple

There are effective health behaviors that remain as yet unproven. But we can't do everything, at least not immediately. Too many choices can be a deterrent to adopting long-lasting change. With massive amounts of information, some of it contradictory and with highly-touted lifestyle interventions vying with each other for incorporation into your daily routine, the high enthusiasm for adopting new health behaviors during this "teachable moment" after breast cancer can actually work against you. One day, you might become a vegan. The next you are prompted to adopt a paleo diet. The next, a macrobiotic diet is the way to go. How do you pick one and stick with it?

This is where we say, keep it simple. There are a lot of good choices out there, but relatively few of them have been validated in medical literature. There are excellent reasons for this. One, it is quite difficult and very expensive to run the types of clinical trials that will prove an intervention is effective. Sometimes, it is impossible to do so. Another, it takes a relatively long time to **prove,** or even to **indicate** that a particular practice, such as a type of diet, is effective. By the time the preponderance of evidence is available for a diet, there are myriad of new ones that have cropped up. Unproven lifestyle habits are not necessarily bad; in fact, they may be very good. However, we choose to focus on those that have a strong track record, so we can be confident and say, doing such and such is proven to improve breast cancer outcomes by X amount. That's where we want to put our energy. We don't want to get distracted by other choices that may or may not be as effective. **The error lies in adopting a health behavior that doesn't help much at the expense of one that does.**

The most effective way to make meaningful change in your healthy lifestyle choices is to narrow it down to the few things that make the most difference. The best way to know for sure is how you feel when adopting specific health behaviors. Do you feel better when you exercise regularly? Do you feel better when you eat well? We will help by leading you to those health behaviors that have been well-validated in medical literature. This book will help you to prioritize so that you can focus your efforts and not get sidetracked by chasing after the next best thing to come around the block. If you want to try new things, by all means, we encourage you to do so, but not at the expense of the basics. In fact, we will prompt you to try new ideas as variations in addition to the basics, in order to keep you from getting bored.

Wellness initiatives need champions

Information motivates. Breast cancer survivors are seeking information. Providing information to breast cancer survivors is highly likely to result in meaningful lifestyle improvements. Yet, it isn't happening often enough. Why? Because wellness initiatives need champions, get very little press, and even less marketing. Yet, this aspect of treatment is just as important. "Big Pharma" can throw a lot of money into sophisticated marketing campaigns promoting a new drug treatment for breast cancer. Academic physicians can become famous for successful completion of a well-performed clinical trial that proves that drug A is better than drug B. We rightfully applaud these advances. But there is no big money or glamour associated with diet or exercise programs.

We all need to become better champions for health behaviors. As patients and as health care providers we need to make the effort to cheer the underdog. We need to emphasize the importance of health behaviors as a component of breast cancer treatment. We believe that wellness practices represent the single greatest unmet need in breast cancer treatment.

Information motivates, but emphasis clinches that motivation and tips it down the path to action. The champions most needed for wellness initiatives are physicians. Patients and nurses are already enthusiastic supporters of wellness initiatives (as evidenced by the number of clinical studies spear-headed by non-physician health care providers and rapid enrollment), but physicians tend to be less outspoken about health behaviors. We believe that this is primarily due to the relatively low profile that wellness studies command in medical literature, and the lack of standard textbooks on the subject. We urge health care providers to become well-versed in the literature related to recommendations that they can make which emphasize the importance of health behaviors. Physicians will then be able to complete their treatment plan with a prescription for wellness that will go farther than imagined in improving outcomes after breast cancer treatment. A major goal of this book is to provide physicians and allied health care providers with the information to make that important step a mainstay of your breast cancer treatment algorithm.

Self-care takes time

If you are like most, even if you have the motivation and desire to change your health habits, there is the looming obstacle of time. Self-care takes time. In the course of this book, we will show you the importance of eating well, getting regular exercise, and practicing mindfulness-based stress reduction. The data is so convincing that we are certain that you will agree that these health habits can truly make an enormous difference in your risk of breast cancer recurrence, and even in your chances of surviving for the next 10 or 20 years.

The real hurdle for most of us is not the decision to change, it's finding the time to incorporate new health behaviors into our lifestyles. Most of the recommendations made throughout this book involve adding another activity into your day. How will you find the time to exercise for 30 minutes per day? How will you carve out 20 minutes of quiet and solitude in the midst of your busy routine? How will you ensure that you not only eat a healthy meal, but take the time to prepare it as well?

Step number one is to commit. If you deem a healthy recovery to be the single most important thing in your life at this point, you will choose to commit one hour per day to that enterprise. The major intent of this book is to present to you the information about how beneficial certain health practices are. Once you see what a big difference **you** can make in your likelihood of surviving breast cancer, ask yourself a simple question: "Am I willing to do what it takes to recover fully, to keep myself in vibrant health, and beat breast cancer?" You've probably already gone through a lot more than it will take from here on out to give you even bigger benefits. But it's not good enough to agree in theory. You must truly commit to lifestyle change. Sadly, as you will see from the data, many breast cancer survivors do not successfully take care of their health. Make sure that you do so by being very clear in your intention and commitment.

Step number two is to become aware of how you spend your time. If there is low-hanging fruit that you use for your down-time, can you make sure that you are using that time to pursue enjoyable but healthy pursuits? Do you sit in front of the television? Replace that time with something more health-conscious. Do you spend your downtime chatting with friends? This is great, and very important, but can you do that while walking together? Take a good look at how you spend every moment of your day, and see whether there are any areas to devote to your self-care.

Odds are, though, that you've already pared your schedule down to the essentials. The problem then becomes that most of us are too busy. Although many of us are masters of efficiency, there is always room to readjust priorities. If your health is more important than other items on your list of daily activities and responsibilities, then one way to ensure that your attention to your health is first is to prioritize it.

This takes practice, because health behaviors aren't usually **demanding** to be done, not like the ringing telephone, or the person who just walked into your office with a problem to solve, or a child to pick up from school **right now**. Make it a practice to put the things that you need to do to keep yourself high up on the priority list. Learn to be OK with saying, "I'll do that right after I finish my meditation." Health coaches and friends can be very helpful with this. Enlist support and establish routines. Remind yourself and everyone around you why these health behaviors are so important. As you make your way through this book, each section will prompt you to establish goals and accountability, and to build up your repertoire.

Carolyn's story

I should be dead by now, I should know. After all, I know breast cancer probably better than anyone else on the planet. I have been at the forefront of breast cancer research and treatment, performing bench-based scientific investigation into the biologic underpinnings of breast cancer, teaching as a Professor of Radiation Oncology at the University level both at home and internationally, leading paradigm-shifting Phase III clinical trials in large co-operative group settings, and treating breast cancer patients in the wonderful multidisciplinary setting at the University of North Carolina's Lineberger Comprehensive Cancer Center. In case that knowledge base wasn't enough, I also learned many lessons from a first-hand experience as I journeyed through surgery, chemotherapy, biological therapy and radiation treatment for my own breast cancer, which kept breaking the rules and coming back to teach me more.

As a scientist, I had intensely studied breast cancer cell biology. Getting breast cancer cells from patients to grow in the laboratory so that we could study what they needed to survive, and therefore how to deprive them of that, was my claim to fame. My specific interest was a newly identified, particularly nasty type of breast cancer, the "triple negative" breast cancer. I was collaborating with the world's experts on triple negative breast cancer when I was diagnosed with one myself. My laboratory was working on strategies to treat triple negative breast cancers, since none of the approaches for other breast cancers were effective. From my laboratory studies, I already knew what didn't work for my type of breast cancer. Somehow, that wasn't very comforting.

The biology bore out. We tried surgery and my breast cancer came back. Next, we tried standard chemotherapy and more surgery. My breast cancer came back. Next, we tried new combinations of biologic agents with chemotherapy. My cancer absolutely loved that and even grew on it. Naturally, more surgery, but even the most aggressive approach couldn't reach all of the cancer. Finally, we turned to radiation therapy.

As a radiation oncologist, I knew all too well that the dose of radiation that we could deliver, even if we exceeded the safe dose, was too low for this tumor. The problem was that I had already received full-dose radiation treatment to that part of my body for treatment of Hodgkin's lymphoma years before. I already lived with significant complications from that treatment, so doubling down on the maximum tolerated dose to the sensitive structures of the nerves, vessels, and lungs was a last resort. Ironically, I wasn't even a candidate for the novel clinical trial that I designed and directed using re-irradiation with a radiation sensitizer, because the dose of radiation that I would need was too high.

We went off-road with something else, under the guidance of the most creative and crazy radiation oncologist in my department. I guess it must have been a heavy load for him to treat his own Chairman, and a breast cancer expert at that, when the stakes were so high.

It was worth a try, but as a breast cancer clinician with years of multidisciplinary breast treatment experience and extensive clinical research under my belt, my colleagues from all around the world and I knew of no one who had survived my particular scenario. I didn't have long to live. It was time to get on with my bucket list.

My husband, 5-year old son, and I boarded our sailboat to sail off into the sunset. Yes, that was a bit risky. I was still very ill. But my husband, Nick, is a physician, and we had everything we needed on board. No treatment options were left at that point, so there was nothing to lose. We were experienced sailors, enough so that Nick could sail single-handily our 38 foot sailboat, *Sweet Carolina*. And, it was on my bucket list.

We didn't think that we would be out for very long, but one day flowed seamlessly into another as we made our way through the islands of the Caribbean, and then South America, and finally Central America. Despite all expectations, I didn't die. I could tell that I still had things going on; I had some enlarged lymph nodes, bone pain, and the expected lymphedema and nerve damage. But as long as I took it easy, I was able to get along. Before we knew it, two years had passed without treatment.

How could this be? I mulled over it. What had I missed? Could we have hit upon just the right combination of chemotherapy, biologics, radiation, and surgery? I doubted that, but clinical trials were investigating that possibility.

There was, however, another possible explanation besides treatment. It was lifestyle. On the boat, we lived simply and healthfully. I spent hours every day gently snorkeling. We ate fish that we caught ourselves, and plenty of vegetables from farmer's markets in parts of the world that didn't use chemicals. Other than the stress of living all together on a small boat and homeschooling our son (the single most difficult thing I have ever done, even though I was a Professor, or maybe because of it), I spent much of my time in peaceful meditation. Could lifestyle have anything to do with my unexpectedly good outcome?

I delved into medical literature with the question: are health and lifestyle factors associated with better breast cancer outcomes? If so, which ones and how effective were they? I was astonished by what I found. And more motivated than ever to continue to do what I could to keep myself as healthy as possible.

I was also chastened by what I felt was a missed opportunity. As a clinician and scientist, I had never realized how effective lifestyle factors can be. The proof was not just personal; the medical literature is quite clear. There are health behaviors that make big differences in breast cancer outcomes. I should have been telling this to all of my patients. I should have been teaching it to my medical students and oncology fellows.

My health didn't permit me to resume my career, but I wanted to continue to do what I could, when I could, to reach out to breast cancer survivors and help to support them, and myself, in maintaining a healthy lifestyle. How to do that, I mused. What did I myself, need for support?

First, the knowledge. In teaching others, I teach myself. I began researching and putting together the information in the form of lectures; after all, that's what I was accustomed to doing.

Second, the practice. It is so difficult to live healthfully in our society. It was much easier on the boat. However, back on land, I needed friends to exercise with me. I needed friends to share healthy meals. I needed kindred spirits and support to keep me on the right path.

That's exactly what I found. A group of like-minded friends, colleagues, and breast cancer survivors put together our ideal support group. It's not your typical breast cancer support group. It's more of a lifestyle practice group, and we call it New Life *after* Cancer. Our goal is to teach and support health practices that have been proven to improve outcomes after breast cancer, and we do so through small-group retreats and workshops.

This book is an amalgam of the information taught in our New Life *after* Cancer workshops and retreats. I hope that you learn as much from this as I have. I can now say with absolute certainty that lifestyle and health behaviors can make an enormous difference in breast cancer outcomes.

Developing awareness

When we started giving lectures and running workshops for New Life *after* Cancer, the first slide said, "Don't gain those post-treatment pounds." It was always point #1, as it is now, because weight gain after breast cancer treatment is so ubiquitous, and so deleterious. It is also a very tough nut to crack, so it deserves our emphasis and attention.

However, we've changed the title. It now says, "Watch out for those post-treatment pounds." It's a subtle, but important difference, one that reflects the entire tenor of our approach. We believe that it's much more effective to try to "do" something than to "not do" something. If we advise you to "don't" do something, that is a negative. Our experience is that it is usually more effective to approach motivational behavior from a positive than a negative view.

Furthermore, to "do" something is empowering. It is an active choice that you make and follow through on. To "don't" do something is an avoidance maneuver. It is motivated by fear more than empowerment, by deprivation rather than actively seeking. Especially when talking about eating or exercising habits, it can be easier to change if you are motivated to do something new as opposed to avoiding a habitual practice. Therefore, throughout New Life *after* Cancer lectures and this book, we won't say something like, "Don't sit on the couch all day watching TV." Instead, we will say, "Make sure that you get, and log, thirty minutes of exercise each day."

There's another reason for the change in title from "don't" to "watch". It is very important to cultivate awareness of our health habits. They are just that, habits. We've been living the same way, typically, since we were young. Rarely have we stopped to look at how we live our lives, and what impact that has on our health and wellness. In order to develop health habits that serve us well, the first step is to take a good look at what we already habitually do.

Eating habits exemplify that concept extremely well. We tend to eat the foods that we grew up eating. If you follow a typical American diet, you probably already know that it is not the best, in terms of health, to say the least. Nutritionists and diet gurus will often say that the single most important aspect of changing your diet is to be aware of what you are eating. Diets that are the most successful (Weight Watchers, to name one) include conscientious notes and logging of what you eat. Step number one of improving your eating habits is to notice, objectively and consistently, what you eat. Develop awareness and watch what you eat.

But we didn't entitle the first part, "Watch what you eat". It is, "Watch out for those post-treatment pounds." They sure can creep up on us. When we encourage you to watch your body for the gradual but inexorable end-results of your health behavior practices, we are getting at something deeper than the day to day reading on a scale. We want to encourage you to cultivate an awareness of changes resulting both from your actions such as, what you eat, how much you exercise, and the results of your health behaviors like how you feel, and how well you maintain your weight.

If you're like most of us, you were probably in a bit of a dazed state with all of the breast cancer stuff going on. It's hard to keep up with everything, let alone keep up with your health maintenance. Good habits like exercise can go by the wayside. It can be hard to eat well if the only thing that tastes good is ice cream. Perhaps you don't particularly want to check in with your body to see how you are feeling. Maybe you feel terrible. Maybe you don't want to invite that feeling in. That's OK. If you're not ready, that's OK. Your mind, your psyche, your body will let you know when you're ready to take charge of your health again. You might not want to read on until you are. We hope you do read on in order to find the motivation and the will to take charge of your health.

Self-Assessment

1) Where in your day can you carve out some time for your own health and wellness? What can you change in your existing regimen to incorporate new health behaviors?

Pull out a piece of paper and go through a typical day, listing what you do and when, as if putting an entry into a calendar. Or do the same exercise on your electronic device.

What can you clip out? What can you delegate? What can you spend less time doing in order to spend time on yourself? Do you have any downtime? When can you squeeze in 30 minutes? Using a calendar, schedule time for **yourself.**

2) What are your impediments to changing health behaviors for the better? Look at your past resolutions. What worked? What didn't? Could you use more motivation? Could you adopt healthy habits that are fun for you? Could you use more support?

Call to Action

This first, and most important step, is straightforward. Simply read on.

But we challenge you to take the plunge: commit to taking care of yourself, to prioritizing your health and wellness. Commit to following this path to wellness.

Pull out a sticky note and declare your commitment to yourself, writing something like, "I will make my health and wellness a priority." Then, post it somewhere prominent, as a reminder to yourself.

Tell three people who are important to your success in making your health a priority that you have made this commitment to yourself.

We will have data-driven calls to action in the following sections. All call to actions rely on your motivation and dedication to adopt healthy lifestyle habits that will improve your outcomes after breast cancer.

PART I:

Watch out for those

Post-Treatment Pounds

Did you know that not gaining weight after treatment is associated with improved survival and reduced risk of recurrence?

Did you know that side effects of treatment, such as lymphedema and hot flashes, are reduced in those that don't gain weight?

Did you know that breast cancer survivors CAN shed those extra pounds, and almost any reasonable strategy works?

Did you know that weight control improves your overall survival outcome?

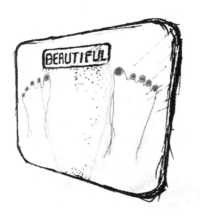

Obesity and breast cancer

Weight control is very difficult to achieve in our society, but its importance for health cannot be overstated. To a large extent, body weight is a composite "read out" of a number of important health practices and lifestyle behaviors. It is also something that virtually all of us are acutely aware of, given that obesity has reached epidemic proportions in many developed nations.

If you are like most, you have struggled with your weight. An important study published in the New England Journal of Medicine showed that Americans gain an average of 3.4 pounds every 4 years. Women gain even more than men (1). It takes motivation and dedication to avoid the seemingly inexorable creep of the pounds. We hope to convince you that weight control is one very important thing that **you** can do to improve your likelihood of a long and healthy life after breast cancer. We will do so by letting the data speak for itself.

The link between obesity and breast cancer outcomes is well-established. The first study to investigate the relationship between weight and breast cancer was published nearly 35 years ago. Quite simply, it showed that women who were overweight had a lower likelihood of survival after breast cancer than those who were not. Since those results were published, many additional studies have examined the relationship between weight and breast cancer prognosis. A review of the pooled data of all of the studies completed before 2005 (a meta-analysis) illustrates the extent of the problem. The results of more than 40 studies show that women who are obese at the time of diagnosis have a 30% higher risk of dying of either breast cancer or other causes than those who are leaner (2).

There are many explanations for why this may be the case. First, women who are heavier tend to have more advanced breast cancer at presentation. Nonetheless, when investigators factor this out by analyzing the data from women with similar disease characteristics, the adverse effect of being overweight still holds, so that is not the only explanation. Second, women who are heavier may also not tolerate treatment as well. Or, more insidiously, may have received relatively lower doses of chemotherapy in the past because of the way that chemotherapy doses are calculated by body surface area instead of weight. At least one well-conducted study indicates that this is the case. The heavier women who received lower relative doses of chemotherapy had an increased risk of recurrence (3). Third, women who are overweight are also at increased risk of other causes of death, such as heart attacks and strokes. Furthermore, their risk of these may be increased with some of the drugs used to treat breast cancer.

There are also biological factors. There is a complicated relationship between body fat and breast cancer that remains relatively poorly understood. You are probably already quite familiar with the fact that the majority of breast cancers express estrogen and progesterone receptors, and also that anti-estrogen treatment such as tamoxifen and the aromatase inhibitor classes of drugs are used to block the growth of breast cancer cells by interfering with these hormonal pathways. Women who are heavier have higher circulating levels of the female hormones that are implicated in breast cancer development and recurrence.

Hormone blocking approaches may also not be as effective in women who have higher levels of estrogen and progesterone. The finding that the deleterious effect of being overweight occurred primarily in women who have estrogen or progesterone receptor-expressing tumors lend credence to this idea (4). Another study to look at the relationship between weight and outcome in breast cancer patients asked specifically about the effect of weight on tamoxifen treatment. The National Surgical Adjuvant Breast and Bowel Project (NSABP) looked at 3,385 patients who had received tamoxifen for lymph node negative, estrogen receptor-positive breast cancer or not. The data from this randomized trial showed that obese women had greater incidence of death compared to normal weight women (5).

Weight control after breast cancer

However, as relevant as the link between obesity and breast cancer may be for those who haven't yet developed breast cancer, it is a moot point for those of us who already have. After all, what can you do now about how much you weighed at the time you developed breast cancer? Regardless of your weight at the time of breast cancer diagnosis, the relevant question after diagnosis is, "Does weight control **after** breast cancer improve outcomes?" The answer is, **yes!**

Before we delve in to the data, there are some common-sense arguments for why you should work toward maintaining a healthy weight that we can draw from the aforementioned studies of the association between weight at diagnosis and outcomes. First, the better outcomes for being leaner are not restricted to breast cancer recurrence. The most important outcome, overall survival, is greatly affected by weight. We know from many, many studies that obesity is deleterious to your health. Unfortunately, the treatments that you may have had to treat breast cancer don't help. In fact, many of the treatments for breast cancer have negative effects on the heart. We will circle back around to this later, but cardiac health is very important for breast cancer survivors, and is clearly linked to obesity. Thus, the data that links healthy weight with better survival still applies to those of us who have already had breast cancer.

A second reason to pay attention to the association between obesity at time of diagnosis and outcomes is that, if you still have your breasts, you are at increased risk for developing another breast cancer. After all, your body has proven that it is capable of allowing breast cancers to grow. Whatever factors influenced the development of the first are probably still in effect now. What does this have to do with weight gain? Well, if you are overweight, the risk of a second breast cancer is even higher. Several studies show an increased risk of breast cancer developing in the opposite breast in heavy women compared to normal weight breast cancer survivors (4, 6).

Another reason has to do with those hormones. Yes, they are important for the risk of getting breast cancer in the first place, but they are also clearly important in helping to keep any lurking residual breast cancer cells from re-growing. After all, that's the whole purpose of endocrine-related treatments such as anti-estrogens and aromatase inhibitors (tamoxifen, anstrazole, etc). For women who had estrogen or progesterone receptor positive breast cancers, reducing circulating hormones is particularly beneficial. It is a well-established fact that overweight women have higher levels of these hormones.

Thus, one can suppose that the associations drawn from the studies of weight at diagnosis and outcomes still apply, even after the fact. The truly motivating question at this point, however, is whether weight change **after** breast cancer diagnosis makes any difference. The Nurses' Health Study asked just that.

Nurses' Health Study: Background

The Nurses' Health study (NHS) is an example of a population-based study, also known as an epidemiological study. It does not involve an intervention. Rather, it asks whether there are associations between one thing and another in a large group of people. The associations are measured by sorting people into groups based on particular factors. In the case of the NHS, the authors grouped women who had breast cancer into categories depending on their weight at the time of diagnosis.

The component of the NHS that looks at whether weight is associated with breast cancer outcomes is actually only one part of a much larger study of many women. 121,700 nurses, age 30-55, agreed to the collection of data on them, on a wide array of factors, including weight, diet, and exercise. Participants filled out detailed questionnaires twice yearly that queried lifestyle and medical history information. The study that is relevant to our discussion is a subset of the larger study.

Of the 120,000 or so women in the NHS, the investigators identified 5,204 women who had developed breast cancer during the course of the questionnaire follow-up. They divided the women into groups based on their weight before diagnosis, as well as categories of weight change after diagnosis. They then looked to see whether breast cancer outcomes were different between the groups.

Of course, they didn't really divide the women into groups. These were data points, and anonymous at that. They divided the data into different groups. They also didn't actually look at weight, rather at body mass index (BMI). This is actually a better measurement for whether someone is overweight or underweight, because it takes into account height, or, more specifically, surface area as determined by height.

Why do these details matter? One, they give a sense for how the data can be handled. There are many different cut-off points that could be chosen to divide the data into different groups. In the case of the study we are discussing, the authors chose categories of <5 kg/m2 BMI loss, maintaining BMI, 0.5-2 kg/m2 gain, and >2 kg/m2 gain. Why? These were probably logical cutoff points for dividing the data into relatively even groups. We don't really need to worry about that, because the reviewers of the study will have done an excellent job of that. We need to be cognizant that when we are extrapolating this data to us as individuals, it does not mean that if you are on the edge of one category, the data in only that category applies to you. These are associations. The actual number doesn't mean as much as the concept.

Two, the specific details of the groupings can be relevant, because they give a flavor of the validity, or at least, of how well the study might apply to you. If you are tall and big-boned and this study measured only weight, you may well say, "It probably doesn't apply to me, because I weigh more but am not overweight." And you would probably be right.

In this study, they got around that by using BMI, a more relevant measurement to pick when categorizing. The point is to encourage you to look at the details of the various studies that we will present throughout this book to see how well they apply to you, personally. Clinicians appreciate a well-designed study that will allow them to extrapolate the results to the majority of their patients, not necessarily to individuals. However, a breast cancer survivor may want to be able to pick and choose those studies that apply most specifically to her unique condition. Our goal is to give enough detail to allow the breast cancer survivor to begin to do this, without being overwhelming. You can choose to skip reading all the details.

We want to emphasize that all of the studies that we will discuss in this and the next few chapters are **indicators**, not crystal balls. Epidemiologic studies such as The NHS point out associations, not cause and effect. They group the data into categories, and statistically query whether a particular event, outcome, or anything else is more likely to be linked to one category than another. Statistics are beyond the scope of this discussion, but suffice to say, associations do not prove a link. However, they can shed a great deal of light on the matter.

Another important factor when evaluating studies published in medical literature is the quality of the journal in which it is published. The most prestigious journals have highly rigorous review criteria. When a study is published in a top journal, you have the benefit of knowing that the world's experts for that particular study have had a hand in questioning and critiquing the findings. This is termed the "peer review" process, and it is extremely stringent; a paper will not be accepted until it meets very high requirements. Almost all of the data that we present is derived from only the top-rated journals. This provides a degree of authority to the results that one doesn't get from the popular media.

The study we are about to discuss Weight, Weight Gain, and Survival after Breast Cancer Diagnosis was published in the Journal of Clinical Oncology in 1995. This is a very well-respected journal, one of the best in the breast cancer field. It is published by the American Society of Clinical Oncology, the premier organization for cancer professionals. The articles published in this journal are subject to a very high degree of professional review by peer experts. When we quote a study from this journal, you can be assured that it is of the highest quality.

Show me the data

In the medical field, when we say that something is **proven**, we are often basing the evidence on the completion of a well-designed, randomized controlled trial. A randomized, controlled trial tests the outcomes of one intervention against another in a group of people with similar disease characteristics. For example, if we wish to see whether a new chemotherapy treatment is better than an established one, the final answer would be determined by a **randomized controlled clinical trial**, where patients with similar type and stage of cancer (or other ways of estimating that they have the same baseline risk of recurrence) are randomly allocated to receive the standard treatment or the new treatment. The outcomes of the two groups (or arms of the trial) are then compared to see whether the result is better with the new treatment.

It takes many years to measure a difference in survival or breast cancer recurrence, but if the results show that the new treatment is better than the old, the new treatment eventually becomes the standard of care. This is how new treatments are tested, and importantly, FDA-approved. This is an oversimplification that doesn't illustrate very well the incredibly long process of testing the new treatment before it even gets to the point of a pivotal randomized trial, nor the level of detail that determines the quality of the trials. The level of evidence derived from a well-performed randomized trial is the highest level of proof.

But there are often cases where a randomized controlled trial simply cannot be performed. Or, as is more often the case, is too expensive or difficult to perform. Lifestyle interventions frequently fall into this category. Instead, health behaviors are often studied by drawing **associations** between the behavior and outcomes. These associations are typically evaluated by large, population-based studies, called **epidemiological studies**. An example of an epidemiological study is one where all of the women diagnosed with breast cancer in a particular region or country during a particular time are asked how much fish they eat on a regular basis. The answers are divided into categories of fish consumption, high or low groups. Then, the incidence of breast cancer recurrence is compared between the high or low groups. If the high-fish consumption group has a lower risk than the low-fish consumption group, then we can conclude that there is an association between fish consumption and breast cancer recurrence risk. Note that this does not prove that fish consumption is causing the reduced risk, because the women weren't randomly assigned to eating more or less fish as the only difference between them. There are many behaviors that go along with particular eating habits, or exercise habits that may be the actual causative factor. However, it is unlikely that a randomized controlled clinical trial will be performed to ask this particular question. After all, if the association exists and the recommendation is readily available and not harmful there is less reason to perform a clinical trial. Do epidemiological studies show proof? No. But the associations that they demonstrate at least help us to know that if we are in a favorable category, we are more likely to have a favorable outcome.

In most cases, we will never have a chance to see the full proof that an association is, indeed, causative. However, there is another way to gain a strong indication of whether or not it might be. Let's jump all the way to the other end of the spectrum from the large, population-based studies. We can turn to the laboratory. Laboratory studies can elucidate mechanisms, the how and why something might work. In the laboratory, we can directly test drug A against drug B. This is done extensively before a clinical trial is even born. The laboratory studies don't necessarily tell us much about how effective the drug may be in real patients, but they do tell us something very important. They tell us how it works, and why. They allow us to manipulate specific conditions so that we can discern cause and effect far better than we can in a complex system like the human body. This can be a very powerful indicator in the case of testing associations discovered in the epidemiological studies. For example, let's take that hypothetical association between fish consumption and risk of breast cancer recurrence. In the laboratory we can directly determine whether the marine fatty acids contained in the fish will inhibit the growth or kill breast cancer cells, and how effectively. Laboratory studies can even tell us how they do so.

By combining the epidemiological study-derived associations with the laboratory study-derived mechanisms, we greatly increase the level of evidence of either alone. If an association is found **and** it is supported by a mechanism that makes sense for why it might have a direct effect on breast cancer outcomes, the likelihood that it is real is much stronger. When randomized clinical trial data is not available, this is the level of evidence that we may use to make decisions about what to do now, as opposed to waiting for the proof that may never make it to trial.

❦ Key Study: NHS

This study asked whether weight before diagnosis or change in weight after diagnosis were associated with breast cancer survival (13). 5,204 women from the larger cohort of 120,000 participants in the Nurses' Health Study developed invasive, non-metastatic breast cancer diagnosis between 1976 and 2000. In these women, BMI was determined both before and >12 months after diagnosis. The data was divided into groups of those who had lost weight, maintained their weight, gained 0.5 to <2 kg/m2 (an average of 6 pounds), or > 2 kg/m2 (an average of 17 pounds). Recurrence rates and survival were determined for each group and compared.

The groups were not even. This is, after all, not a randomized trial. Women who gained weight after diagnosis tended to be younger. Women who gained the most weight tended to have more advanced disease, and to have received treatment with chemotherapy or tamoxifen. These differences were taken into account by multivariate analysis. In other words, the potential differences in outcomes between groups that could be due to imbalance of factors other than weight change were handled statistically to remove the influence of the other factors in order to look specifically at weight change.

The study showed that weight gain was associated with an increased risk of recurrence, death due to breast cancer, and overall death. Women who gained an average of 6 pounds had a 40% increased risk of breast cancer recurrence compared to those who maintained or lost weight. Women who gained more than an average of 17 pounds had a 53% increased risk of recurrence.

With regard to survival, women who gained weight after treatment also had a correspondingly higher risk of death overall, as well as death specifically due to breast cancer.

There was roughly a 35% increased risk of both breast cancer death or any death for those who gained a modest amount of weight. The increase in risk was even higher for those who fell into the highest category of weight gain, around 60% for both breast cancer death and death from any cause.

An interesting caveat, however, was that the increased risk associated with weight gain was only seen in women who didn't smoke. Due to finding a difference in the relationship between weight and outcomes in non-smokers as opposed to smokers and age, the investigators separated out the results based on smoking and menopausal status. Presumably, smoking is driving outcome factors more strongly than weight.

A striking finding was that the women who started out closer to a normal weight and gained even a modest amount of weight after breast cancer diagnosis comprised the group in which the adverse association between weight gain and recurrence was the strongest. The investigators postulate that additional weight gain in those who are already heavy may not influence disease characteristics beyond those that are already in play; we already know that the risk is higher for more overweight women. However, for those who are not overweight at the time of diagnosis, gaining those post-treatment pounds may make a greater difference in outcome.

♀ Key Study: CWLS

The Nurses' Health Study raised a flurry of debate because earlier studies that looked at weight change after diagnosis had not found a very strong association between weight gain and breast cancer outcomes. However, since the publication of the NHS, a growing body of data suggests that a higher risk of recurrence and death is indeed associated with weight gain after diagnosis. Furthermore, the increased risk is not necessarily restricted to specific groups, such as those who are non-smokers or less overweight at the time of diagnosis.

Let's look at a report from the Collaborative Women's Longevity Study (CWLS). The CWLS was an observational study of nearly 4,000 women with breast cancer who lived in New Hampshire, Massachusetts, or Wisconsin. Participants completed a structured telephone interview after diagnosis and returned a mailed follow-up questionnaire, on average about 5 years after they had been diagnosed with breast cancer. Investigators then followed the outcomes of these women to see whether various health behaviors correlated with breast cancer recurrence risk or death. One of the questions asked was whether weight change after breast cancer diagnosis was associated with breast cancer recurrence or death.

The study found a strong correlation between weight gain and risk of death from either breast cancer or any cause (14). In fact, for every 5 kg weight gain after diagnosis (roughly 10 pounds), there was a 13% increase in the risk of dying from breast cancer. Furthermore, there was an even higher increased risk, 19% of dying from heart disease.

The theme of heart disease will be a recurring one as we look at breast cancer outcomes. Cardiovascular disease is the number one killer of women in the United States. Furthermore, several breast cancer treatments can exacerbate the risk of cardiovascular disease. Radiation, doxorubicin (Adriamycin) and trastuzumab (Herceptin) are the main culprits. For breast cancer survivors, attention to cardiac health goes a long way toward overall survival.

The CWLS study illustrates that point. During the course of an average of 6.4 years of follow-up, when one would expect most of the breast cancer recurrences to occur, there were only slightly more deaths from breast cancer than there were from cardiovascular disease.

The results of the CWLS study corroborate and extend the findings of the NHS. But not all studies agree. Another large study did not find an increased risk of death from breast cancer and weight gain (15). However, that study looked at weight gain only in the first year of diagnosis, not over the longer time span of the other studies. Furthermore, the study had many fewer "events" to report, meaning that it may have lacked the statistical strength to identify an association. As with many lifestyle interventions, it may be that the duration is very important.

♀ Key Study: Long Island Study

The Long Island Breast Cancer study did an excellent job of looking at weight over time. This study recruited nearly 1,500 women from Long Island, NY who were diagnosed with breast cancer between 1996 and 1997. Weight at various times after breast cancer diagnosis was recorded. When the investigators compared weight one year before, at diagnosis, and one year after diagnosis, as well as further time points, they were able to get a very accurate picture of how weight changes over time relate to breast cancer outcomes.

Consistent with the findings from the NHS and the CWLS, the Long Island study showed that women who maintained their pre-diagnosis weight did significantly better than those who gained more than 10% of their body weight after diagnosis (16). The effect was quite striking; women who gained a significant amount of weight had **more than 2.5-fold increased risk of dying, from either breast cancer or from other causes of death.** We emphasize: watch out for those post-treatment pounds!

The risk from weight gain appeared to be stronger if the gain occurred soon after breast cancer diagnosis (within the first 2 years). It also was just as pronounced for women who started out heavy as for those who started out non-overweight. (You may recall that the NHS showed the highest risk in those who had normal weight before diagnosis but then gained weight). There was also a suggestion that the risk of a worse outcome may be higher in younger women who gain weight than in older women, similar to the NHS study.

Weight control improves side effects and complications

Weight control is not just about improving survival; there are also other excellent reasons to avoid weight gain after treatment. Being overweight affects how one feels and has an influence on some very important breast cancer related health issues. In other words, weight control is also relevant to reducing the risk of breast cancer complications.

The Healthy Eating Activity Lifestyle (HEAL) study looked at breast cancer related symptoms in women after breast cancer treatment (18). The investigators asked whether weight was associated with a number of breast cancer outcomes.

Not surprisingly, women who were overweight (BMI >30 kg/m2) had poorer overall physical functioning. However, it is interesting to note that a number of cancer-related symptoms were higher in those who gained more than 5% of their body weight compared to those who did not, including worse lymphedema. Furthermore, the HEAL investigators found that women who lost weight after breast cancer treatment had less chest wall and arm pain than those who gained weight after treatment (19).

The link between weight and lymphedema had already been established, but the HEAL study confirmed that association. Perhaps more importantly, a randomized controlled trial was performed to ask whether weight loss would improve lymphedema (20). In this small but relevant study, 21 women with breast cancer-related lymphedema were randomized to a weight reduction coaching program or general dietary advice (the control arm). The women in the weight reduction program did achieve weight loss compared to the women in the control arm. The women in the weight reduction program had a significant reduction in lymphedema by the end of the 12-week program compared to those who did not receive the weight reduction program. While we look forward to the validation of this study by additional studies, this randomized controlled trial provides important evidence that weight loss is an effective strategy for reducing lymphedema.

Being overweight is also linked to hot flashes. More than half of breast cancer survivors develop hot flashes as a result of treatment. Hot flashes interfere with sleep, work, and quality of life. The Women's Healthy Eating and Living (WHEL) study investigators asked whether weight change after breast cancer was associated with the frequency or severity of hot flashes (21). Breast cancer survivors who gained more than 10% of their pre-diagnosis weight after treatment were a third more likely to have hot flashes than those whose weight remained stable. Avoiding weight gain after diagnosis may be an effective way to reduce hot flashes.

Can weight loss post-diagnosis improve outcomes?

In aggregate, the data strongly suggest, but do not prove, that gaining weight after breast cancer is bad for breast cancer survivors. Of course, to prove this, we would need to see a randomized controlled clinical trial. And we simply don't have results from such a trial at this point. Nor are we likely to have one. The benefits of avoiding weight gain from a non-breast cancer standpoint are already so well-established that it would seem to be a moot point to design and carry out a trial that asks whether weight gain after breast cancer is bad.

The relevant question now is whether weight **loss** after breast cancer is beneficial. Unfortunately, we don't have a clear answer to this question yet. We do, however, have some strong clues as to what that answer will be.

The CWLS indicates that, while weight gain is to be avoided, weight loss is not necessarily associated with improved survival. It wasn't only those who gained weight after breast cancer who fared worse; the study found that weight loss was also associated with an increased risk of death (albeit not from breast cancer). Similarly, the Long Island study found that women who lost more than 5% of their body weight after breast cancer fared worse. These data caution against more than modest weight loss after diagnosis.

However, it is important to note that the weight loss may not have been intentional. It is quite likely that the women who lost weight had intercurrent health problems or other cancers that were responsible for both the weight loss and the worse outcomes. If you are otherwise healthy, there is no evidence that losing weight intentionally is harmful from a breast cancer standpoint. However, it is worth noting that weight loss was **not** associated with a reduced risk of death from breast cancer in this study.

Of course, the clearest way to determine whether weight loss is beneficial is to test that question directly in the context of a controlled clinical trial. This is particularly important when one considers all of the health benefits of not being overweight, and would resolve the question as to whether other causes were driving the findings of the CWLS and Long Island studies.

The Lifestyle Intervention Study Adjuvant (LISA) trial was designed to provide the answer we seek. The LISA study was a multi-center randomized controlled clinical trial that asked whether obese breast cancer survivors who were being treated with letrozole, an endocrine therapy, would have better outcomes if they lost weight. Three hundred and thirty women were enrolled; half were randomized to a telephone-based weight loss intervention that provided diet and exercise coaching, the other half received usual care.

The first important finding from this study was that the weight loss goals **were** achieved in the intervention group. Women in the intervention group lost at least 5% of their body weight within 6 months, and maintained on average a 3.6% decrease in their body weight for a year (17). This, in itself, is a very significant result. It underscores that weight loss **is** achievable in breast cancer survivors. Indeed, breast cancer survivors seem to do better than most when compared to other weight loss studies. This is particularly notable when one considers that the intervention was a readily-accessible telephone-based coaching regimen. It is inexpensive to deliver and easy to expand to all breast cancer survivors.

However, while the participants in the study did their part, the pharmaceutical company that was sponsoring the trial did not. Funding was yanked before the outcomes were available. We will not have the answer from this trial. What a tragedy!

A similar study, the Exercise and Nutrition to Enhance Recovery and Good Health for You (ENERGY) trial has shown that overweight breast cancer survivors can lose weight, and we are awaiting the answer as to whether this improves outcomes. It will be many years before we have the answer from this trial. That is, we will if it doesn't get scrapped like the LISA trial did. If you are overweight, you can wait for the results, which we all suspect will show that reducing weight to a healthy level improves breast cancer outcomes as much or more than maintaining weight does.

Or, you can get started now and be at a healthy weight by the time we have the proof. After all, we already know that being overweight worsens some other important outcomes, such as breast cancer treatment complications, physical functioning, and even overall quality of life.

So where does that leave us? **Watch those post-treatment pounds.** If you (or your patients) are just finishing treatment, the data is clear that not gaining weight is associated with improved survival and reduced risk of recurrence. If you gained weight after breast cancer, getting back to your pre-treatment weight is likely to be beneficial. You will feel better without the extra pounds, you won't have the effects of that added fat, and you will fall into the category of women with the best outcomes. However, don't overshoot it. More may not be better.

Weight or waist?

Is it just weight that matters? Probably not. If you'd like to delve into the science, read the next section. If you want to skip the details, the bottom line is that it's the abdominal fat cells that are the main suspect. But not all fat is bad. After all, our bodies need fat. We also need muscle. We need everything in a good balance.

When we gain fat above and beyond what the body needs, it puts the extra fat somewhere. In all too many middle-aged women, the fat goes around the belly. Unfortunately, this abdominal fat tends to be quite metabolically active with all of the things that we don't want the fat cells to produce.

A number of studies have recently looked into the ramifications of excess abdominal fat. Stated another way, they ask, "Which is more relevant - the weight or the waist?" In one study by the HEAL investigators, they measured waist circumference and waist-to-hip ratio in breast cancer survivors to see whether breast cancer outcomes differed between curvaceous and round women (22). They also looked at fat-related metabolic factors - insulin, glucose, C-peptide, IGF-1 and binding protein-3, C-reactive protein, and adiponectin.

After nearly 10 years, the study found that a round body habitus (higher waist to hip ratio) was associated with a risk of both breast cancer recurrence-induced death and death from any cause. There was a 4-fold increased risk of breast cancer recurrence-related death in women who were the rounder, and women with larger waist circumference had a 3-fold increase in death from any cause. However, it is also important to note that the risks occurred only in those women who were the largest/roundest. Women with a waist circumference of more than 99 cm (go ahead, get your tape measure and check) and a waist circumference to hip ratio of >0.83 were the ones with the increased risk.

Another study confirmed these findings. The California Breast Cancer Consortium also found that a larger waist to hip ratio (roundness, not curvaceousness) was related to risk of death (23). This is consistent also with other large studies that show increased risk of death in women (and men) who didn't have breast cancer who had larger waist circumference (24).

These studies support the idea that the real target of weight control strategies should be to reduce the excess abdominal fat. Overall weight, or BMI, may be a surrogate for gauging how much metabolically active fat one carries. If so, weight loss, per se, may not be as effective as toning. Thus, exercise may be a critical component of any weight control strategy.

Biology: What's so bad about fat?

The human body is an amazing biological system. It is beautifully complex, and yet, when we look into specific reasons for why things work (or don't) the way they do, we can often get a glimmer of how it all falls together, of how it makes sense. You may find it helpful to learn more about the fascinating underlying biology affecting the growth of breast cancer cells.

In its simplest terms, cancer is a problem of growth control. Cancer cells are our own body's cells that have learned to ignore signals to stop growing or that have been stimulated to grow inappropriately. Treatment of cancer often focus on killing cancer cells, but it can be just as important, and potentially as effective, to stop the growth of cancer cells. Particularly when treatment is finished, understanding what helps to keep cancer cell growth under control becomes very important.

Most of the lifestyle factors that we will discuss do just that. They change the environment of the body to favor tumor control. Lifestyle factors are the ultimate "biological" treatment, because they influence the entire organism - both tumor cells and normal cells.

In reality, we understand very little about tumor biology. We understand even less about whole-organ (whole person) biology. But if we look at what may be going on at a cellular level, to the tumor cells and normal tissue environment, it all begins to make a much clearer picture.

Let's start with fat. We just discussed the link between breast cancer and obesity. What are some of the biological underpinnings for that link? And what relevance does that have to breast cancer recurrence risk or survival after breast cancer treatment? What's so bad about fat? After all, our bodies need a healthy balance of fat. However, not all fat cells in our bodies are the same; in fact, they are quite different. The adipocytes (fat cells) in the waist and belly region are metabolically active. These belly fat cells are called "central adipocytes", and they are factories for several powerful breast cancer cell growth stimulators.

One such factor is adipokine. Adipokine promotes the production of inflammatory factors. Inflammation creates a strong tumor-promoting state. The concept of "silent inflammation" is well-known for its effects on cardiac health, but it is also a state that is very conducive to breast cancer development and growth. We use the term "state" to emphasize that inflammation creates a whole environment. There are individual inflammatory factors that can directly stimulate breast cancer cell growth, but it is the overall environment produced by inflammation that is probably more important than any individual factor. The inflammatory factors that adipocytes produce in response to the adipokine secreted by belly fat cells have been shown to stimulate breast cancer cell growth, but also, perhaps more importantly, stimulate remodeling of the extracellular matrix to create an environment that is favorable for tumor development and growth (7).

Two inflammatory mediators that are directly linked to breast cancer recurrence, C-reactive protein (CRP) and interleukin 6 (IL-6), are produced by central adipocytes. Both have been correlated with worse outcomes in breast cancer survivors. In fact, the Glasgow Prognostic Score, which predicts survival in women with metastatic breast cancer, incorporates CRP and other inflammatory mediators that are produced by adipocytes in the model (8). Higher levels of CRP have been associated with a doubling of the risk of recurrence and death (9).

Leptin is another protein produced by centrally located adipocytes. It is elevated in obese women. Leptin stimulates angiogenesis, the formation of new blood vessels that tumors need to be able to grow beyond a certain size. Leptin also activates insulin-like growth factor 1 (IGF-1), a powerful breast cancer growth factor that will come up as an important target in many of our discussions of the different lifestyle interventions (10, 11).

Adipocytes in normal weight women secrete another factor, adiponectin, which counteracts the tumor-promoting leptin, to keep things in check. Leptin is necessary for normal breast development, and adiponectin tells it when to turn off. However, this adiponectin, the negative regulator of leptin, is decreased in obese women. Furthermore, levels of adiponectin are inversely related to the risk of developing breast cancer, meaning that the higher the levels of "good" adiponectin, the lower the likelihood of being diagnosed with breast cancer (12). Thus, the fat cells from obese women are promoting inflammatory mediators and tumor growth factors, while those from normal weight women are kept in check by balancing factors such as adiponectin.

Inflammation is just one part of the equation, and we will discuss inflammatory mediators more in later chapters. But fat cells also contribute to other factors that are important in breast cancer development, such as estrogen and other sex hormones involved in breast cancer development and growth.

Estrogen is a very potent growth factor for the majority of breast cancers. Most of the body's estrogen is made in the sex organs (the gonads) in premenopausal women. However, the adrenal glands also produce a small amount of sex hormones, in the form of precursors. A precursor has to be processed in order to become active, and that's what fat cells can do for estrogen and other female sex hormones. This source of estrogen is particularly important after menopause, when it becomes the main supply of female sex hormones.

Studies show clearly that heavier women, particularly heavier postmenopausal women, have increased levels of estrogens compared to leaner women. Furthermore, sex hormone binding globulin, an inhibitor of one of the principal estrogens, estradiol, is reduced in heavier women. This factor binds to and sequesters estrogens (hence its name "binding globulin), effectively removing them from the general circulation. Heavier women have less of this inhibiting factor. And, just to add insult to injury, estrogens up-regulate leptin expression, leading to further imbalance in the pro-breast cancer promoting factors. Being heavier makes more estrogen which makes more leptin, creating a combination of powerful pro-tumor factors.

How can breast cancer survivors lose weight?

If you are convinced by the data that we have to date, and feel that it is in your best interest to trim down if you are overweight, no doubt your next question will be: "How?" If you are a health care professional, the major barrier to discussing the importance of weight control with your patients may be the inherent difficulty in answering that question. It may also be the well-founded belief that it won't make any difference if you do recommend weight control, because studies in the general population show that 95% of your patients will not "listen". But it doesn't really have to be so difficult, and it is certainly not "hopeless".

We can turn to the recent and ongoing clinical trials to answer the question of how best to approach weight control in breast cancer survivors. Let's briefly review them with an eye to the methods these studies employed to achieve healthy weight loss.

In the LISA trial that we just discussed, participants in both the intervention and the control group received information in the mail to teach about public-health recommendations for healthy diet and physical activity (17). They also received a 2-year subscription to the Canadian Health Magazine. It is notable that the women in the control group, the ones who received no additional counseling, successfully maintained their weight; they did not **gain** weight. Remember, the data shows that not gaining weight is already associated with significant improvements in breast cancer outcomes. Thus, at the very least, **do** read and take to heart the American Cancer Society recommendations for exercise and diet. They are based on solid evidence. And reinforcing that message with your favorite health magazine seems to work very well.

The intervention in the LISA trial went a step further, though, and added a 2-year telephone coaching program. The coaches had specific goals: lose 1-2 pounds per week until a 10% weight loss was reached (as long as above a BMI of 21). They recommended: cutting calories to 1250-1750 kcal/day, reducing fat intake to 20% of total calories, and increasing fruits/vegetables and grains. There was also a physical activity requirement of 150-200 minutes of moderate exercise per week. Doesn't this sound like just about any reasonable weight loss program you may have investigated?

The coaching consisted of about 20 sessions. The calls were frequent during the first month, and then tapered down until they occurred once every 3 months in the second year. The telephone conversations were reinforced by information that was sent to summarize the content of each call. In addition to checking on diet and exercise, the coaches also helped to identify and overcome behavioral patterns and beliefs that appeared to be barriers to successful weight control as well as improve coping skills.

The FRESH START trial showed that 543 breast and prostate cancer survivors could lose and keep off 2-3% of their body weight (25). In this trial, participants received materials aimed at increasing exercise, fruit and vegetable intake, and decreasing dietary fat. The intervention arm received a workbook and a series of six newsletters delivered every seven weeks and personally tailored on type of cancer, cancer coping style, race, age, self-efficacy, stage of readiness, and barriers and/or progress toward goal behavior. The goal was to get at least 30 minutes of exercise 5 days per week, 5 or more servings of vegetables and fruit per day, and 30% or less of total calories from fat. As with the LISA trial, this trial proved that high quality information is effective motivation.

The Healthy Weight Management trial was designed to determine the effect of a cognitive behavioral therapy (CBT) intervention for weight loss through exercise and diet modification. Eighty-five overweight or obese breast cancer survivors were randomly assigned to a once weekly, 16-week intervention or wait-list control group. The study used an approach that was specifically designed for the needs of obese women, addressing a reduction in energy intake, as well exercise, with a goal of an average of one hour per day of moderate to vigorous activity. The results showed significant differences in weight and body fat indices in the women who were randomized to receive the intervention compared to those who did not, with an average of 8% weight loss after one year (26).

Another trial, the Reach out to Enhance Wellness in Older Survivors (RENEW) trial used a mailed instruction and telephone counseling intervention in elderly long-term survivors of breast, prostate, and colorectal cancer. The intervention group had an average weight loss of 3%, sustained over a 2-year period (27).

Are you seeing a pattern here? Overweight breast cancer survivors can, indeed, lose weight. Even if they were never successful before. It takes dedication and motivation, but when better to start than when the stakes are so high. The studies all have three things in common. They all use 1) high quality information with specific instructions, 2) exercise, and 3) good eating practices. That is exactly what we are going to focus on for the next few sections of the book.

We wish that we could finish out this section with the answer of whether or not these effective weight-loss approaches improved breast cancer outcomes, but we can't. We don't have those answers yet. But we will, as these studies mature. Until then, know that breast cancer survivors **can** lose weight, using simple and reasonable approaches.

How about dieting?

Note that none of the trials we've discussed touted a specific type of diet. They focus on generally good eating habits (and exercise - don't forget that component!). There are, however, a few studies that do look specifically at the effects of low-fat, low-carbohydrate, or high-vegetable and fruit diets. We will discuss these in greater detail in following chapters, but we would like to briefly touch on two of them now that specifically highlight weight loss as their main focus.

The first is a randomized, controlled trial that compared a low-fat versus a reduced-carbohydrate diet to determine whether one or the other was better with regard to weight loss for overweight breast cancer survivors who were receiving adjuvant hormonal treatment (28). Both approaches resulted in effective weight loss, and to a similar degree. Furthermore, both diets improved metabolic markers that are associated with better health outcomes (29). The low-carbohydrate diet was expected to improve insulin-related metabolism, which it did, but so did the low-fat diet. Conversely, the low-fat diet was expected to improve lipid profiles, which it did, but so did the reduced carbohydrate diet. Similar studies are ongoing, but at present it seems that almost any reasonable diet strategy will do the trick.

The second is the Women's Interventional Nutrition Study (WINS). This randomized, controlled clinical trial asked whether breast cancer survivors who followed a very low-fat diet would have better outcomes than those who followed a standard diet (30). We will get into the full details in Part III, but the short answer is, yes, they did. However, the debate about the results of this study continue because we don't know whether the benefit was a direct result of reducing fats (the primary question of the study) or an indirect result due to the weight loss that occurred in the low-fat group. Since the low-fat diet group lost weight and the regular diet group did not, this trial has been considered the best proof that we have to date that weight loss is associated with better breast cancer survival. Some would even go as far as to say that this trial constitutes the proof we seek that weight loss is responsible for the improved survival.

It seems that just about any diet works, as long as it is well-balanced, targets modest weight loss, and includes exercise. A group of investigators is currently testing just that: what if you allow breast cancer survivors to choose their own diet style, low-fat or low-carb? Guess what. It works. Breast cancer survivors who self-selected either diet lost weight compared to a control group that was assigned to neither diet (31). It doesn't really matter what you choose. It matters that you do it. In fact, the investigators of this trial looked specifically to see whether the higher amounts of fat consumed in the low-carb diet were deleterious. They found no evidence that lipid levels were adversely affected. Conversely, the fasting glucose and insulin levels were not adversely affected in the low-fat but consequently higher carb diets. The answer for both physicians and patients is quite simple. Anything will do, and any reasonable diet seems safe.

Prescription: Part I

Maintain a healthy weight

The evidence:

- A meta-analysis of more than 40 studies shows that women who are obese at the time of diagnosis have a 30% higher risk of dying of either breast cancer or other causes than those who are leaner.
- The Nurses' Health Study (NHS) showed that breast cancer survivors whose body mass increased after diagnosis were at increased risk of both breast cancer recurrence, death from breast cancer, or death overall. An average weight gain of six pounds was associated with a 1.4-fold increased risk of recurrence, and higher weight gain (average of 17 pounds) with 1.53-fold increased risk of recurrence. Risk of death was increased 1.6-fold in the group with the highest weight gain. Those who started out at a healthy weight but then gained weight after diagnosis had the strongest association between weight gain and breast cancer recurrence.
- The Collaborative Women's Longevity Study (CWLS) demonstrated a 13% increased risk of dying from breast cancer with each 5 kg weight gain after diagnosis. The increased risk of death due to heart disease was even higher.
- The Long Island study found that breast cancer survivors who gained more than 10% of their body weight had a greater than 2.5-fold increased risk of dying from either breast cancer or other causes.

- The Healthy Eating and Living Study (HEAL) found that 5% weight gain was associated with lymphedema, while weight loss was associated with less lymphedema and chest wall pain.
- The Women's Healthy Eating and Living (WHEL) study found that more than 10% weight gain was associated with increased hot flashes.
- While several trials demonstrate that weight loss is feasible, we await results to determine whether weight loss improves outcomes.

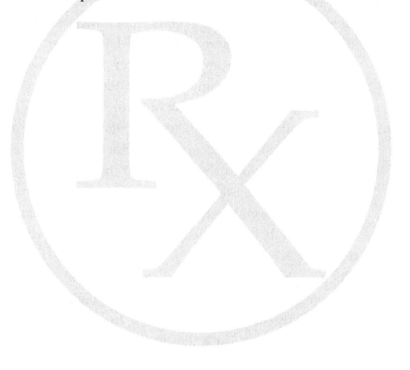

Lolly's weight loss story

I was an overweight kid who was put on my first doctor's diet at age six. During my public school years, sometimes I was plump and sometimes not. I have a stocky, muscular body type and I am only 5' 1 ¾" tall. By high school, I was pretty much at average weight. In college, sometimes I was thin and sometimes not. As an adult I struggled with my weight, trying many, many diets. I often lost weight successfully, but gradually I would gain back the weight I had lost and more. During my early 50's, I eventually weighed 212 pounds. Clearly, I was obese! I dieted and lost 65 pounds and never regained all of that weight. But at the time of my breast cancer diagnosis, I had gained back more 20 pounds.

After recovery from the mastectomy, I had an appointment with my internist who just happened to mention that a friend of hers was a radiation oncologist and a breast cancer survivor who told my doctor that the best thing one could do to avoid recurrence was to not gain weight, so she challenged me to lose 10 pounds. That friend was Carolyn Sartor. So, I knew Carolyn long before she knew me!

Another friend introduced me to New Life *after* Cancer and I was a participant in its second retreat with Carolyn, a fabulous cruise to the Caribbean. During the retreat, participants were encouraged to set goals for themselves, and I did so. I committed to lose that 10 pounds my doctor mentioned and to start taking yoga. I began taking yoga and dieting the same day in March 2010. I used Dr. Mike Moreno's *17 Day Diet*, which worked very well for me. I lost 10 pounds the first month and thought that was pretty easy, so I committed to lose another 10, and then another 10 and then five pounds for a total of 35 pounds within three months. I am at a very comfortable weight for me.

I had to get a complete new wardrobe which was fun, and I feel so much better. Not only that, but it is wonderful to know that I am increasing my chances for longevity and helping to avoid a recurrence of breast cancer. I have kept off that weight for four years, but it is not easy! I set for myself a 10-pound range, and when I get to the top of that range, I go back on a weight loss program until I am again at or near the bottom of that range. I wish I were able to lose weight only once and be done, but my personal weight history predicts that that is not going to happen with me. I have to stay on top of maintaining a healthy weight and I have committed to do so. And I still practice yoga four times a week.

Self-Assessment: Part I

How do you measure up?

You may not have really looked at what your weight has become after treatment. After all, dieting is often the last thing on our minds during chemotherapy, or even possibly for several years after treatment. Yet, for most of us, the pounds may have accumulated more than we like, and more than is good for us.

The first place to begin is to see clearly just where you are, before even considering whether you might wish to tip the balance in your favor. To do so, follow these steps to fill out the chart below.

1. Step on a scale and determine your weight today.

2. For the pre-diagnosis weight, use your typical weight during the timeframe of a year before diagnosis.

3. To find the change in weight, find the difference between the two weights.

4. To find the percent change in weight, subtract the weight before diagnosis from the current weight, then divide that number by the weight before diagnosis and then convert to a percentage by multiplying that number by 100. Presumably, your height hasn't changed.

5. To calculate your BMI, go to a BMI calculator site: http://www.nhlbi.nih.gov/health/educational/lose_wt/BMI /bmicalc.htm and enter your weight and height for both now and before diagnosis. The calculator will give you your BMI in units of kg/m2.

6. Finally, determine the change in your BMI from before to after treatment.

Self-Assessment

1. Weight today =	
2. Pre-diagnosis weight =	
3. Change in weight =	
4. % Change in weight =	
5. Height =	
6. BMI today =	
7. Pre-diagnosis BMI =	
8. BMI change =	

Now you can use your **BMI change** info and see where you fall with regard to the data that we have discussed by finding your specific cell in the tables below from the Nurses' Health Study.

BMI change	RR death	RR brca death	RR recurrence
-0.5	1.11	1.01	0.99
Maintain	1.0	1.0	1.0
+0.5-2	1.35	1.35	1.40
>2	1.59	1.64	1.53

RR stands for "relative risk", which means the risk compared to a given group, in this case the group that maintained their weight. Thus, a relative risk for death of 1.59 means that women whose body mass increased by more than 2 kg/m2 after diagnosis have 1.59 times the risk of death than women who maintained their weight after diagnosis. Likewise, brca death means death due to breast cancer.

Use your weight change in the next table from the Collaborative Women's Longevity study.

Weight change	HR death	HR brca death	CVD death
Lose 22+ lbs	2.66	0.64	1.08
Lose 22-4 lbs	1.39	0.90	1.02
Maintain	1.0	1.0	1.0
Gain 4-13 lbs	0.98	0.98	0.79
Gain 13-22	1.06	1.28	0.64
Gain 22+ lbs	1.70	1.78	1.73

The risk is quoted as a "hazard ratio", abbreviated as HR. This is very similar to relative risk, but calculated over time as opposed to one time-point. For our purposes, the relative risk and hazard ratio can be thought of as the same, as both connote the degree of increased risk compared to a reference group (those who maintained their weight). This is why the "maintain" column will always show 1.0; that is the reference group.

Note that the relative risk or hazard ratio can be less than 1, as in the case of the risk of breast cancer death for women who lost more than 22 pounds after diagnosis. The hazard ratio of 0.64 for this group means that their risk of dying from breast cancer is only 64% of the risk of the reference group (those who maintained weight). Thus, a hazard ratio or relative risk of less than 1 means that the group is at lower likelihood of breast cancer recurrence-induced death. This shows that the higher risk of death in women who lost weight after diagnosis is not due to breast cancer, but due to other causes (albeit not cardiac. CVD stands for cardiovascular disease)

Finally, you can use your **percent weight** change to estimate your risk based on the Long Island Study.

Percentage weight change	HR death	HR brca death
>5% loss	5.3	7.25
Maintain	1.00	1.00
5-10% gain	1.08	0.84
>10% gain	2.72	2.80

You may have noticed that the different studies gave you different risk assessments. This is normal to have differences between studies, and emphasizes the point that these are estimates, and not exact numbers. However, this exercise will serve to let you have a general idea of how motivated you want to be based on your own individual situation.

Call to Action: Part I

Watch out for those post-treatment pounds! Whether your self-assessment showed that you are right where you want to be or indicated that you could improve, it starts with developing awareness.

The "homework" for this section is simple. Weigh yourself every day. Then, write that weight down in a notebook so that you can track it. (I suggest that you get a notebook that you can use to track various health behaviors as they are introduced in this book. By the end, you will be able to see how much you have improved your lifestyle!)

It sounds simple, but it can be deceptive. Many of us have barriers to overcome when it comes to acknowledging how much we weigh. It can be frustrating and downright discouraging if you are unhappy with the scale's answer. But keep it up. The discipline of tracking, that is, of observing and recording, is one of the most effective single actions you can undertake on your journey toward a healthier lifestyle. If you are not ready to do that, to consistently check your weight each day and record it, you are probably not motivated to take on this particular change right now. That's OK. There's a time for everything. If that's the case, move on to another part that appeals to you.

If you want to take it a step further and do more than merely observing your weight, the next few chapters will lead you gently down a path of exercise and healthy eating that will help you to maintain an optimal weight for your body. You may be motivated to start a diet right now. We don't want to discourage the enthusiasm, but perhaps you could start by defining your support structure. What

Call to Action

encourages long-term, sustainable change for you? Whether it be friends or a health coach to share the journey, identifying habits that don't serve you well in favor of those that do, or finding time to exercise, put some thought this week into building the structure that works for you.

In the next few parts, we will delve into the data that supports specific exercise and eating recommendations. You will find this to be very helpful when choosing between one weight loss strategy and another. So, before you pick a diet to begin, read on.

References: Part I

1) Mozaffarian D, Hao T, Rimm E et al. Changes in diet and lifestyle and long-term weight gain in women and men. NEJM 2011; 364: 2392-404.

2) Protani M, Coory M, Martin JH. Effect of obesity on survival of women with breast cancer: systemic review and meta-analysis. Breast Cancer Res Treat 2010; 123:627-35.

3) Rosber G, Hargis J, Hollis D, et al. Relationship between toxicity and obesity in women receiving adjuvant chemotherapy for breast cancer: results from CALGB Study 8541. J Clin Oncol. 1996; 14:3000-8.

4) Sparano J, Want M, Zhao F, et al. Obesity at diagnosis is associated with inferior outcomes in hormone receptor-positive operable breast cancer. Cancer 2012; 118:5937-46.

5) Dignam J, Wieand K, Hohnson K et al. Obesity, tamoxifen use, and outcomes in women with estrogen receptor-positive early-stage breast cancer. JNCI 2003; 95:1467-76.

6) Li C, Malone K, Porter P et al. Epidemiologic and molecular risk factors for contralateral breast cancer among young women. Br J Cancer 2002; 89:513-8.

7) Champ C, Volek J, Signlin J et al. Weight Gain, Metabolic syndrome, and breast cancer recurrence: are dietary recommendations supported by the data? Int J Br Ca 2012; 3:1-9.

8) Al Murri A, Bartlett J, Canney P et al. Evaluation of an inflammation-based prognostic score (GPS) in patients with metastatic breast cancer. Br J Cancer 2006; 94:227-30.

9) Pier B, Ballard-Barbash R, Bernstein L et al. Elevated biomarkers of inflammation are associated with reduced survival month breast cancer patients. JCO 2009; 27:3437-3444.

10) Garofalo C and Surmacz E. Leptin and cancer. J cellular Phys 2006; 207:12-22.

11) Cirillo D, Rachiglio A, LaMontagna R et al. Leptin signaling in breast cancer; an overview. J Cellular Biochem 2008; 105:956-64.

12) Grossmann M, Ray A, Dogan S et al. Balance of adiponectin and leptin modulates breast cancer cell growth. Cell Research 2008; 18:1154-56.

13) Kroenke C, Chen W, Rosner B et al. Weight, weight gain, and survival after breast cancer diagnosis. J Clin Oncology 2005; 23:1370-78.

14) Nichols H, Dietz A, Egan K et al. Body Mass Index before and after breast cancer diagnosis: associations with all-cause, breast

cancer, and cardiovascular disease mortality. Cancer Epidemiol biomarkers Prev 2009; 18:1403-9.

15) Caan B, Kwan M, Hartzell G et al. Pre-diagnosis body mass index, post-diagnosis weight change, and prognosis among women with early stage breast cancer. Cancer Causes Control 2008; 19:1319-28.

16) Bradshaw P, Ibrahim J, Stevens J et al. Postdiagnosis change in bodyweight and survival after breast cancer diagnosis. Epidemiology 2012; 23:320-27.

17) Goodwin P, Segal R, Vallis M et al. Randomized trial of a telephone-based weight loss intervention in postmentopausal women with breast cancer receiving letrozole: The LISA trial. J Clin Oncol 2014; 32:2231-39.

18) Imagyama I, Alfano CM, Neuhouser M et al. Weight, inflammation, cancer-related symptoms and health related quality of life among breast cancer survivors. Breast Cancer Res Treat 2013; 140:159-76.

19) Paskett E, Dean J, Oliveri J et al. JClinOncol 2012; 30:3726-3733.

20) Shaw C, Mortimer P, and Judd P. A randomized controlled trial of weight reduction as a treatment for breast cancer-related lymphedema. Cancer 2007; 110:1868-74.

21) Caan B, Emond J, Su H et al. J Clin Oncol 2012; 30:1492-97.

22) George S, Bernstein L, Smith A et al. Central adiposity after breast cancer diagnosis is related to mortality in the Health, Eating, Activity, and Lifestyle study. Br Ca Res Treat 2014; 146:647-55.

23) Kwan M, John E, Caan B et al. Obesity and mortality after breast cancer by race/ethnicity: the California Breast Cancer Survivorship Consortium. Am J Epidemiol 2014; 179:95-111.

24) Pischon T, Boeing H, Hoffmann K et al. General and abdominal adiposity and risk of death in Europe. NEJM 2008; 359:2105-20.

25) Demark-Wahnefried W, Clipp E, Lipkus I et al. Main outcomes of the FRESH START trial: a sequentially tailored, diet and exercise mailed print intervention among breast and prostate cancer survivors. J Clin Oncol 2007; 25:2709-18.

26) Mefferd K, Nichols J, Pakiz B et al. A cognitive behavioral therapy intervention to promote weight loss improves body composition and blood lipid profiles among overweight breast cancer survivors. Breast Cancer Res Treat 2007; 104:145-52..

27) Demark-Wahnefried W, Morey M, Sloane R et al. Reach out to enhance wellness home-based diet-exercise intervention promotes reproducible and sustainable long-term improvements in health behaviors, body weight, and physical functioning in older, overweight/obese cancer survivors. J Clin Oncol 2012; 30:2354-61.

28) Thompson C, Stopeck A, Be a J, Cusslr E, Nari E, Frey G, and Thompson P. Changes in body weight and metabolic indexes in overweight breast cancer survivors enrolled in a randomized trial of low-fat vs. reduced carbohydrate diets. Nutrition and Cancer 2010, 68:1142-52.

29) Thompson H, Sedlacek S, Paul D et al. Effect of dietary patterns differing in carbohydrate and fat content on blood lipid and glucose profiles based on weight-loss success of breast-cancer survivors. Breast Cancer Research 2012; 14:R1.

30) Chlebowski R, Blackburn G, Thomson C et al. Dietary fat reduction and breast cancer outcome: interim efficacy results from the Women's Intervention Nutrition study. J National Cancer Inst 2006; 98:1767-76.

31) Sedlacek A, Playdon M, Wolfe P, et al. Effect of a low fat versus a low carbohydrate weight loss dietary intervention on biomarkers of long term survival in breast cancer patients ('CHOICE'): study protocol. BMC Cancer 2011; 11:287-297.

Part II: Exercise

Did you know that exercise reduces your risk of breast cancer recurrence and death?

Did you know that it only takes a modest amount of exercise to see those benefits and more?

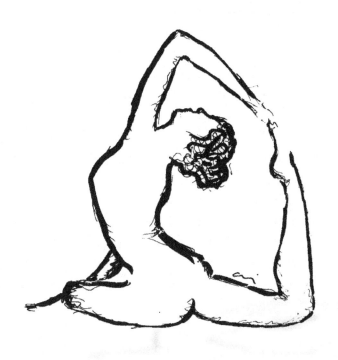

Exercise and breast cancer

If you asked us to choose only one lifestyle practice to recommend after breast cancer, we would pick exercise. Exercise is the single most important goal because it provides so many beneficial outcomes. We discussed the importance of weight control in the preceding chapter. Exercise certainly helps with that. It not only helps you to convert calories into action, but it also promotes healthy metabolism. In fact, exercise can compensate for less than optimal eating habits. Exercise also makes you feel good. It improves mood and overall quality of life. It helps to keep your entire body functioning well, overcoming side effects that may be a result of treatment, such as fatigue or lymphedema. Finally, exercise reduces the risk of breast cancer recurrence and improves survival.

Investigators at the National Cancer Institute reviewed all of the data on exercise and breast cancer published by 2012 (1). They looked specifically for studies that asked the question of whether exercise was associated with breast cancer recurrence or survival. They excluded studies that combined exercise with diet, so as to focus specifically on exercise. They found 17 studies that looked at whether exercise either before or after diagnosis was associated with breast cancer-specific survival or overall survival.

In the next few sections, we will take a close look at a few of the eight studies that looked specifically at exercise **after** diagnosis. However, we can summarize the findings by quoting the National Cancer Institute investigators directly: "There is fairly consistent evidence that physical activity either before or after breast cancer diagnosis is associated with a reduction in both breast cancer-specific mortality and overall mortality." Another expert states it more succinctly. In his review of the literature on the influence of diet and exercise on breast cancer incidence and outcome, Rowan Chlebowski states, "Perhaps the lifestyle factor most strongly and consistently associated with both breast cancer incidence and recurrence is physical activity" (2). Let's look at the data.

⚲ Key Study: NHS

Studies show that physical activity is associated with a lower risk of developing breast cancer. A summary of the data estimates a 20-40% lower risk of developing breast cancer in more active women (3). Similar to weight, however, the relevant question for breast cancer survivors is not whether exercise **before** diagnosis makes a difference in outcomes, but whether exercise **after** diagnosis does. The investigators of the Nurses' Health Study (NHS) that was discussed in Part I were the first to ask the question of whether exercise **after** diagnosis was linked to breast cancer survival.

As you may recall, the NHS was a large epidemiological study of over 120,000 nurses. To ask whether exercise is associated with breast cancer outcomes, the investigators turned to the data of the nearly 3,000 women in the study who had developed breast cancer, and who had provided information about their exercise habits, including how much, how often, and how intense the exercise. Exercise was scored in terms of Met-hours/week, which is a way of giving a common unit to various forms of exercise. The average amount of exercise after diagnosis was 9 Met-hours per week, the equivalent of walking at a moderate pace for a total of three hours per week.

The results showed a clear benefit to exercise after diagnosis (4). Breast cancer survivors who engaged in at least 3 Met-hours of exercise per week had significantly lower risk of death from breast cancer and death from any cause compared to those who exercised less than 3 Met-hours per week. Exercise was associated with a 40% reduced risk of dying from breast cancer, and 35% reduced risk of dying from any cause.

These are substantial and significant improvements. The 10-year survival for women who engaged in more than 3 Met-hours per week was 92%, as opposed to 86% for those who exercised less than 3 Met-hours per week. To emphasize how important these results are, ponder this for a moment: Women who got the equivalent of one-half hour of walking per day had a 6% **absolute** reduction in death compared to those who didn't exercise. This means that six out of every 100 breast cancer survivors could have their lives saved by moderate exercise.

If we see benefits of this magnitude from chemotherapy or radiation, it's considered a home run, paradigm shifting, the big news plastered all over the front page of the news. Granted, the NHS is not randomized controlled trial data; it is not "proof" that exercise is the direct cause, the only factor at work here. Nonetheless, after dedicating entire professional careers and cancer hospitals to trying to get results like this, it is astonishing that every breast cancer survivor doesn't get out and exercise. The association with better outcomes is **strong**; the magnitude of the benefit is **enormous**.

There's even more good news. It didn't take all that much exercise to see the benefits. Women who exercised at least

3 Met-hours per week did just as well as those who exercised more than 9 Met-hours per week, compared to those who got little or no exercise. In other words, walking at an average pace for one hour per week was enough to see an effect, while walking for three hours per week puts one securely in the benefit zone. It also didn't require an intense workout to get the benefit. Walking or other forms of moderate exercise appeared to be just as effective as running, or more intense exercise.

The benefit of exercise was particularly apparent in women with hormone-responsive tumors. This supports that hypothesis that exercise may exert its beneficial effect through reduction of estrogen hormone levels. Finally, the benefits of exercise were seen regardless of BMI or obesity. Everyone benefitted, indicating that exercise may help to overcome the negative effects of being overweight discussed in Part I.

Leveling the playing field for exercise

Activity is a difficult thing to measure. After all, the energy used when running full speed is very different from that used when playing a game of golf. Yet, both are forms of effective exercise.

In order to report the data in a way that can evaluate different forms of exercise in a "common currency," a standard measurement is needed. One such measurement of exercise is the Met. Met stands for "metabolically equivalent task," defined as the ratio of the metabolic rate associated with each activity divided by the resting metabolic rate. One Met is the energy expended while sitting quietly. Walking at a moderate pace is assigned 3 Mets, jogging is 7, and running is 12. Running hard uses about four times more energy than walking. In this manner, different forms of exercise are assigned different metabolic activity levels, or Mets (5).

With exercise, the amount of time also affects the energy used. Thus, time is factored in by reporting exercise as Met-hours. Walking for one hour is measured as three Mets x one hour, or 3 Met-hours. If you walk for two hours, it would be 3 Mets x 2 hours, or 6 Met-hours.

In this manner of reporting, exercise units become interchangeable. For example, running for 15 minutes is equivalent to walking for one hour. The Met-hours system helps to calibrate the exercise into an interchangeable unit that can be compared across different forms and duration of exercise. You can look up Met values for specific activities and calculate your own exercise to see which results apply to you at the Self-Assessment at the end of this chapter.

♀ Key Study: CWLS

Another study corroborates the findings of the NHS. Like the NHS, the Collaborative Women's Longevity Study (CWLS) was an epidemiological study of health behaviors over time in a particular cohort of breast cancer survivors. Women who had been recently diagnosed with breast cancer (cases) or women who were similarly matched for factors such as age (controls) completed a telephone interview within two years of diagnosis that asked about lifestyle practices. The investigators asked whether various health behaviors were associated with outcomes in the breast cancer survivors.

The study examined the relationship between exercise after breast cancer diagnosis and risk of dying from breast cancer in nearly 4,500 women who completed a follow-up survey questionnaire after the initial telephone interview asked specifically about exercise (6). The median time from diagnosis to the time of survey completion was 5.6 years. Fewer than 10% of participants were less than two years from diagnosis, while 13% were more than 10 years from diagnosis at the time of enrollment in the study. Reported exercise was quantified by Met-hours/week and the data divided into four even categories, which turned out to be <2.7 Met-hours/week, 2.8-7.9 Met-hours/week, 8.0-20.9 Met-hours/week, and >21 met/hour week.

A moderate amount of exercise (defined as >2.8 Met-hours/week) was associated with a significantly lower risk of dying from breast cancer - a 35% lower risk, to be exact. These results confirm the findings from the NHS.

The investigators of the CWLS study found something that the NHS had not seen. Breast cancer survivors who exercised more saw more benefit. Those who exercised 8 – 20.9 Met-hours/week had a 41% lower risk of dying from breast cancer, while those who exercised more than 21 Met-hours/week had a 49% lower risk. While these reductions in risk are fairly similar across the groups, meaning that the majority of the benefit is seen with modest exercise, there was a statistically significant trend to suggest that more is slightly better. The investigators calculated that each increase of 5 Met-hours/week lowered the risk of breast cancer death by 15%.

Data was collected an average of five years after diagnosis, so this study looks at exercise habits over a longer time span after diagnosis than some of the other studies. This allowed the investigators to query whether the timing of exercise, early after diagnosis or picked up later, made a difference. It might relieve those of us who became motivated to exercise a few years after diagnosis to note that the results showed that physical activity resulted in an important benefit on survival regardless of the interval since breast cancer diagnosis.

Another pearl from this study relates to the type of exercise. The investigators asked whether the intensity of the exercise made a difference, that is, whether higher Met exercise as opposed to Met-hours of exercise was related to outcomes. To some extent, this is captured in the calculation of Met-hours equivalents, but the question of intensity relates to biology behind the effectiveness of exercise; vigorous exercise results in different biological processes than modest exercise. The CWLS investigators found that moderate exercise was just as effective as vigorous exercise.

The results of this study are **very** encouraging. It doesn't take much exercise to see a significant benefit. Furthermore, the exercise doesn't have to be terribly difficult. Finally, there's no time like the present to get going with your exercise plan. The benefits persisted even if exercise didn't begin right away after diagnosis.

⚷ Key Study: HEAL

Another important study asked specifically whether a change in exercise after diagnosis was related to outcomes of breast cancer survivors.

The HEAL study was designed to investigate the association of a number of lifestyle factors on breast cancer outcomes. This study enrolled more than 1,100 women who were diagnosed with breast cancer, as opposed to the NHS that enrolled healthy women and then identified those who had developed breast cancer during the course of the study. The ability to look at changes over time is an advantage of a **prospective** study, such as this one. Specifically, participants were asked about physical activity in the year before, and two years after diagnosis. The investigators successfully collected pre- and post-diagnosis exercise information on nearly 700 participants (7). They looked at changes in pre- to post-diagnosis exercise levels, and whether this correlated with whether or not women in different exercise categories were more or less likely to survive their breast cancer.

By now, it won't surprise you to see that the study showed a clear benefit in survival for those who exercised. Women who engaged in at least 9 Met-hours per week of exercise (equivalent to walking for 3 hours each week) **before** diagnosis had a 31% lower risk of death compared to inactive women. The benefits of exercise were even greater when focusing on exercise habits **after** diagnosis, however. Breast cancer survivors who were active in the two years after diagnosis **reduced their risk of death by two-thirds** compared to inactive women.

This study provides a wonderful opportunity to see the effects of changing exercise patterns after diagnosis. The good news is that even if you were inactive before diagnosis, if you exercise afterward you may be at significantly lower risk of death. The HEAL study showed that women who were inactive before diagnosis and then picked up their exercise after breast cancer had a **45% lower risk of death**.

In case that wasn't enough to motivate you, here's another statistic. But be forewarned, this one is chilling. Women who exercised regularly before breast cancer, and then dropped their exercise habits after diagnosis were **four times more likely to die.** Take that with a grain of salt, because there are many reasons that women who are no longer able to exercise are in ill health. It could be a life-threatening illness (besides breast cancer) that induced them to stop exercising. The HEAL investigators also found that the women who decreased their physical activity after diagnosis gained more weight than the women who increased their exercise. As discussed in Part I, keeping those post-treatment pounds down is associated with better outcomes.

If, like many of us, you perhaps became a bit of a slug after the rigors of treatment, let these results cause you to sit up and commit to getting back in shape! If you are just finishing up your treatment, these data show that exercise after breast cancer is one of the most effective things that you can do to improve your likelihood of survival.

♀ *Key Study: WHI*

Here's another study that looked specifically at change in exercise levels from before to after diagnosis. The Women's Health Initiative (WHI) studied exercise habits of more than 4,600 breast cancer survivors, comparing pre- and post-diagnosis exercise levels. The assessment was at either three or six years after diagnosis, so later than the assessment in the HEAL study.

This study confirmed the others. Breast cancer survivors who exercised nine or more Met-hours/week after diagnosis had a **39% lower risk of death** from breast cancer, and **46% lower chance of dying** from any cause (8). With regard to change in exercise habits after diagnosis, it is encouraging to note that 40% of breast cancer survivors in this study increased their exercise levels after diagnosis, while 35% maintained their pre-diagnosis activity levels. Women who increased or maintained physical activity to the 9 Met-hours/week level had 33% lower risk of death. This was true even for those who were inactive before diagnosis.

Exercise provides a prime example of how the diagnosis of breast cancer can lead to the motivation of health habits that can improve your outcomes even beyond those that are breast cancer related. You may not ever have been a very active person. But now, armed with the information that gentle exercise program can reduce your risk of breast cancer as much or more than anything else you can do, you may well be motivated to do what you have never done before. Importantly, the exercise program that you start today will not only reduce your risk of breast cancer recurrence, it will improve your cardiac and pulmonary health, your metabolism, your mood, and your overall quality of life.

♀ *Key Study: WHEL*

Not all of the studies show that increasing activity after breast cancer diagnosis is associated with improved survival. One that did not is the Women's Healthy Eating and Living (WHEL) Study. Let's look to see what we can learn from that.

95

The WHEL study was a randomized controlled clinical trial that asked whether a low-fat diet would improve breast cancer outcomes (9). We will discuss the main study in detail in a later chapter that focuses on diet, but let's look now at a side study that the investigators performed using the data from the WHEL trial.

Of the 3,000 participants in the larger study, there was data on 2,300 who had completed a questionnaire about activity at both baseline and one year after diagnosis and who had not had a recurrence by that time. The investigators asked whether baseline exercise or change in exercise between baseline and one year after diagnosis was associated with outcome.

Before looking at the conclusions they draw from this specific question, there are some interesting and important caveats. First, only half of the participants were getting the recommended amount of exercise either at baseline, or, sadly, even one year after diagnosis. Considering that this is a group that was voluntarily participating in a healthy lifestyles program, this statistic is very disappointing. Furthermore, of those 1,100 or so women with breast cancer who were not meeting the minimum exercise recommendations, more than three-fourths continued to to get insufficient exercise one year later. Indeed, only 213 women who were not regular exercisers increased their exercise to the minimum recommended amount.

So even before examining the results, it is important to understand that this study contained only a small proportion of participants who actually fit the question that we are asking: does a modest increase in exercise after diagnosis make any difference? Thus, it is not surprising that the investigators did not see a strong association between **change** in exercise habits and breast cancer outcomes.

They did, however, see a clear benefit from exercising. Women who exercised regularly before diagnosis had a third less likelihood of death than those who did not meet the exercise guidelines. Outcomes were even better for those who exceeded the recommended amount of exercise; women who did the equivalent of at least an hour of brisk walking five days per week had 50% less risk of death compared to those who exercised minimally. Furthermore, there was the suggestion that the benefit of exercise comes from sticking with it. Women who met the physical guidelines at both baseline and one year were at decreased risk of death (mostly from breast cancer) than those who weren't getting the recommended amount of exercise at baseline or at one year after diagnosis. In other words, to those of you who are regularly exercising, keep it up!

How does this study compare to the HEAL study, which showed that women who were inactive and then increased their activity after breast cancer did so much better? One important difference between the studies is the duration of time after diagnosis/treatment. In the WHEL study, investigators looked at one-year change in activity. In the HEAL study, investigators were querying longer-term exercise habits (two to three years after diagnosis) (10). Indeed, all of the studies that we discussed have looked at exercise patterns over a longer timespan than did the WHEL study.

The take home message that we can apply from this study is that it is important to keep with your exercise program.

The short-term benefits may not be as remarkable as the long-term benefits. This is a very important factor to consider when it comes to motivation. Just as with a weight-loss diet, an exercise program can be easy to start, but much more difficult to continue. Gym memberships certainly use that aspect of human nature to their advantage! So, although this may be a negative study, when taken in context with the other studies, it provides a very important point that we should take to heart.

♀ Key Study: ABCPP

Does getting the minimum recommended exercise really make that much of a difference? The After Breast Cancer Pooling Project (ABCPP) asked that question. The U. S. Department of Health and Human Services recommends engaging in at least 2.5 hours per week of moderate intensity exercise (10 Met-hours/week). The After Breast Cancer Pooling Project put together the data from more than 13,000 breast cancer survivors to ask whether meeting this recommended amount of exercise made a difference in outcomes after breast cancer.

Yes, breast cancer survivors who engaged in at least 10 Met-hours per week of exercise had a 25% reduction in the risk of dying from breast cancer, and a 27% reduction in the risk of dying from any cause (11). The benefits were even greater at higher levels of exercise. Moderate levels of exercise are consistently linked to improved survival after breast cancer.

Sadly, many breast cancer survivors do not get enough exercise. The ABCPP findings were the same as other studies discussed; less than half of breast cancer survivors are getting the minimum amount of recommended exercise. **Half!** We can do better than this!

♀ Key Study: A meta-analysis of published studies

We've discussed several, but not all, or the studies related to exercise in breast cancer survivors. Let's round out the data by looking at a meta-analysis of all of the studies performed as of 2010 (12). In total, eight studies were identified, of which six were included in the meta-analysis. Four of those directly addressed the question of post-diagnosis exercise, in a total of more than 10,000 breast cancer survivors.

The results allow us to better quantitate the benefit of exercise across different studies and different groups of women. The investigators found that exercise after diagnosis significantly reduced the risk of breast cancer recurrence (by 24%), the risk of death due to breast cancer (by 34%), and the risk of dying from any cause (by 41%).

The various studies used different exercise cut-off points, but the investigators of the meta-analysis tried to statistically smooth out the junctions to see whether they could determine different outcomes based on more or less exercise. They defined low level exercise as less than 2.8 Met-hours/week, intermediate as 2.8 – 8.9, intermediate-high as greater than 8.9, and high as more than 15. Each of these levels of physical activity showed a significantly reduced risk of dying from breast cancer compared to those who got low or no exercise.

Do these data prove that exercise reduces the risk of breast cancer death? Not necessarily. To do that would require the results of a randomized clinical trial. However, we don't yet have the results from randomized clinical trials to give us that proof. Fortunately, there are several trials that are currently ongoing so we shouldn't have to wait too long. In the meantime, however, we will leave you with this conclusion of the data we have to date: moderate exercise after diagnosis is strongly associated with reducing breast cancer deaths.

Seeing the forest for the trees

It can be all too easy to lose sight of the big picture in focusing on the detailed results of individual studies. In fact, one can sometimes get lost when one study seemingly contradicts another. Sometimes, the clearest answer emerges from looking at a group of similar studies as a whole, instead of one by one.

That is what a "meta-analysis" does. A meta-analysis is a statistical approach that is used to combine the data from a number of similar trials. This effectively smooths the road, evening the bumps and dips between one study and the next to provide an overall answer. A meta-analysis uses much more data than that available from a single trial, and thus has the power to detect whether a relatively small benefit is "real." It also useful for determining just how effective an intervention is when results of some of the studies are significantly better than others. The meta-analysis provides the global view from a large number of smaller perspectives.

How is a meta-analysis performed? Investigators identify all of the studies that have been performed to answer a particular question. In this case, that would be all of the studies of exercise in breast cancer survivors. They don't leave any of the studies out so as not to introduce a selection bias. However, they do look at each study to determine the quality, and low quality studies are discounted or de-emphasized. They create a larger dataset by pooling the data from the individual studies, and then use this metadata to compute the results.

Thus, in order to perform a meta-analysis like the one we discussed for exercise, one first needs a question that has been answered by a decent number of individual studies. The purpose of the meta-analysis is to gain clarity, to put the results of those trials into a global perspective. Importantly, a meta-analysis provides not only the proof that something works, but also a quantitative measurement of just how well it does so. This is called the **effect size**, which can then be used to compare how effective one intervention is compared to another. The higher the effect size, the more effective the intervention.

Biology: How does exercise work?

There are several ways in which exercise might work to improve breast cancer outcomes. Some of those mechanisms are related to the ones we discussed in the first chapter.

Estrogen hormones: Circulating estrogens are potent growth factors for estrogen/progesterone-expressing breast cancers, and the effect of exercise on reducing estrogen hormone levels is well established in healthy young athletes. But does moderate exercise reduce estrogen levels in breast cancer survivors, many of whom are already postmenopausal? The answer is yes. A randomized trial of exercise among overweight postmenopausal women showed that exercise reduced levels of estrogen (13). Thus, one very likely explanation for the effect of exercise on breast cancer recurrence is a reduction in estrogen. This is supported by the finding in many of the studies of exercise and breast cancer that the benefit of exercise appears to be stronger in women with hormone-receptor positive breast cancers.

Insulin signaling pathways: Exercise, through its effects on the insulin signaling pathways, may also improve breast cancer outcomes in women whose tumors do not express estrogen. We will discuss insulin signaling in more detail later, but for now suffice to say that insulin-like growth factors can be potent stimulators for some of the estrogen-receptor negative tumors, like the "triple negative" breast cancer subtypes. Exercise helps to drive glucose into cells, thereby reducing the amount of insulin necessary to accomplish this goal. Thus, physical activity reduces insulin resistance and hyperinsulinemia that are related to worse outcomes in breast cancer survivors (14, 15, 16, 17, 18). Further, a randomized clinical trial of breast cancer survivors showed that exercise reduces insulin-like growth factors and increases insulin-like growth factor binding proteins, effectively reducing these tumor growth factors (19).

Inflammation: One of the points we touched on in the last chapter is equally relevant here: reducing the risk of cardiac disease in breast cancer survivors. It is worth noting that the benefits of exercise are equally strong for improving overall survival, not only breast cancer survival. Exercise is well known to improve cardiac health. One of the mechanisms by which it does so may be equally relevant to breast cancer recurrence; exercise reduces inflammation. We discussed in Part I that C-reactive protein (CRP), a global marker of inflammation, is strongly associated with breast cancer outcomes. A randomized controlled trial showed that exercise training reduced levels of CRP in breast cancer survivors (20). Note that this randomized trial can elucidates cause and effect, not only associations. It is well known that elevated CRP is associated with cardiac disease (it is an independent cardiac risk factor). It is also clear that higher CRP levels are associated with worse breast cancer outcomes (it is an independent breast cancer risk factor). And it is now known that exercise reduces CRP levels in breast cancer survivors. Can you connect the dots?

Immunity: You may have noticed that the same mechanisms that we discussed in Part I have come into play again, namely, estrogenic hormones, insulin-like factors, and inflammation. Let's introduce another mechanism: immunity. Our body's immune system is ever vigilant in seeking and destroying cancer cells that may be lurking in the dark corners. You can think of it like a police force, trying to keep law and order. With a full-strength force of NK cells (natural killer cells), any stray cancer cells will be neutralized. But if our immune function is depleted, that force isn't as effective. The informative randomized trial of exercise in breast cancer survivors that shed light on exercise's role in improving insulin metabolism and inflammation also proved that exercise improved immune function in breast cancer survivors (21). Kudos to the investigators of the Rehabilitation exercise for health after breast cancer (REHAB) trial and to the participants in that trial for providing such insight into just how exercise might be exerting its influence on breast cancer outcomes.

The effect of exercise on immunity might also explain why high levels of exercise may not be better than moderate. Very intense exercise performed frequently can actually lower immune function. Just as losing too much weight too quickly can be counterproductive, stressing one's body with too much physical activity can also be bad; all things in moderation.

Exercise during treatment

Now you know the benefits of exercise **after** diagnosis and treatment, but what if you are currently undergoing breast cancer treatment? Should you wait until it is all done, risking the reconditioning and difficulty of getting back into shape? Or should you carry on with exercise during treatment? What about starting an exercise program during treatment if you are highly motivated by the data already presented?

Some may be deterred by a fear that exercise during and after treatment might not be safe. However, in 2010, the American College of Sports Medicine reviewed the research on the safety and effectiveness of exercise during and after treatment and found that not only was exercise safe, but also that there were improvements in physical function, quality of life, and cancer-related fatigue, among other things (22).

There is an excellent study that sheds light on the subject of exercise **during** treatment. The Supervised Trial of Aerobic Versus Resistance Training (START) study was a randomized clinical trial performed in Canada (23). The investigators asked whether quality of life was improved by exercise during chemotherapy for breast cancer. A second question was whether aerobic or resistance exercise (strength training) offered different benefits.

Between 2003 and 2005, 242 breast cancer patients who were beginning their chemotherapy treatment were randomized to a usual care/non-exercise program or an aerobic exercise program or a strength-training program. It is interesting to note that only 33% of all people who were offered enrollment in the study decided to participate. If you were offered a free training program during chemotherapy, would you take it? We hope so! Those who decided to participate did an excellent job of following through with the entire 17-week program, whether aerobic or resistance exercise.

The most important take away from this study was that exercise was well tolerated during chemotherapy. While quality of life scores were higher in the exercise groups than the non-exercise control group, they were not significantly better overall. Several other parameters were improved by exercise, however. Aerobic exercise improved self-esteem, fitness, and lowered body fat percentage. Resistance exercise also improved self-esteem, but also muscular strength and lean body mass. In other words, exercise helped chemotherapy recipients to feel better about themselves and to have healthier bodies.

This translated into an unexpected, but very important effect. Women who were randomized to the strength-training exercise program were more likely to be able to complete a full-dose chemotherapy course. Additionally, they did so needing fewer hematopoietic support drugs. In other words, a stronger body resulted in being better able to tolerate the chemotherapy. This is a profoundly important finding. However, it was not the primary question of the study, so there must be further investigation into the effect of exercise on treatment tolerance to confirm these results.

Prescription: Part II

Exercise

The evidence:

- The Nurses' Health Study (NHS) showed that women who engaged in more than 3 Met-hours per week (e.g., walked the equivalent of one or more hours per week) had 40% lower risk of dying from breast cancer and 35% lower risk of death from any cause. The 10-year survival for breast cancer survivors who engaged in more than 9 Met-hours/week of moderate exercise was 92% vs 86% for those who exercised less than 3 Met-hours/week, a 6% absolute survival benefit (4).

- The Collaborative Women's Longevity Study (CWLS) confirmed and extended the NHS findings of a benefit of exercise even at the lower level of 3 Met-hours/week, but also found additional improvement with more exercise, but not with more intense exercise. The investigators calculate that each increase of 5 Met-hours/week of exercise lowered the relative risk of breast cancer death by 15% (6).

- The Healthy Eating and Living (HEAL) study looked at change in exercise habits 2 years after diagnosis. Women who exercised after diagnosis reduced their risk by two-thirds. Even those who were inactive before diagnosis reduced their risk of death by 45% if they exercised after diagnosis. In contrast, those who had originally been active but then stopped exercising after diagnosis had a four-fold increased risk of death (7).

- The Women's Health Initiative Study (WHI) confirmed the findings of the HEAL study that an increase in exercise after diagnosis is associated with improved survival. Those who exercised 9 or more Met-hours/week after diagnosis had a 39% lower risk of death from breast cancer and 46% lower risk of dying from any cause (8).

- The After Breast Cancer Pooling Project (ABCPP) polled 13,000 breast cancer survivors and found that less than **half** were meeting the U.S. Department of Health and Human Services recommendation for 10 Met-hours/week of exercise. Those who did meet the minimum had a 25% reduced risk of dying from breast cancer and 27% reduced risk of dying from any cause (11).

- A meta-analysis of eight post-diagnosis exercise studies quantified the benefits. Exercise above 3 Met-hours per week reduced the risk of breast cancer recurrence by 24%, or death due to breast cancer by 34%, and of death due to any cause by 41% (12).

- The Supervised Trial of Aerobic Versus Resistance Training randomized trial showed that exercise during chemotherapy is not only safe and well tolerated, but improved self-esteem and physical parameters. Aerobic exercise improved fitness and percentage of body fat, while resistance exercise improved strength and lean body mass. Interestingly, resistance exercise also improved chemotherapy completion rates (23).

Alice's exercise story

I'm not one who loves to wake up and pound the pavement at 5 o'clock in the morning; I'd rather enjoy watching the *Today* Show with a nice cup of coffee before heading out to my office. Perhaps that is why I've always struggled with my weight?

When I was in my late 30s, I was invited to play tennis with a group of women who were putting together a night tennis league team. Even though I'm fairly athletic, I'd been sedentary since college and the last time I'd played tennis was in high school! My racquet was made of some material that is non-existent now and my game was one straight out of the 1970's. That first season was a disaster and I think I developed more blisters and bruised egos than anything else. Still, I decided that getting back on the tennis court was going to be the best way of getting back into the world of exercise.

I decided to take some individual tennis lessons and slowly, I joined in on some group lessons and clinics. I bought modern tennis gear, complete with an updated racquet and tennis shoes that weren't the flimsy old Tretorns of days-gone-by. I met some other women who were getting back into tennis and we formed our own tennis team. I'm happy and proud to say that I still play tennis with most of those women and when I was diagnosed with breast cancer, they were some of my most ardent supporters. They even had T-shirts made that read: Breast Friends Make the Best Tennis Buddies.

By the time I was diagnosed in December of 2009, I was playing tennis regularly and doing some type of additional exercise, but not nearly to the extent that I enjoy in my life today. While I was in treatment, I didn't do very much in the way of "real" exercise during the first few rounds of chemotherapy (Adriamycin Cytoxan). I regularly attended my tennis team's matches and so cheering them on was my best and most fun form of exercise. Later, as I finished the Taxol chemotherapy treatments, I started to get back into some light exercise. I began some individual sessions with Lauren, a wonderful personal trainer and tennis professional who has since become a good friend. She'd worked with another person who had been treated for breast cancer and through Lauren's encouragement; I began to get back on the treadmill and onto the floor with various core exercises. I also began playing what I referred to as "lite tennis" with friends who didn't care about the level of play, but were there for the enjoyment.

Two important things happened to me as a result of the breast cancer diagnosis. I became part of a study at UNC called "Get Real and HEEL" and in the study, I worked with a personal trainer on exercise and I also worked with a therapist on mindfulness. The other wonderful thing that happened was that I met Carolyn Sartor, the former Chief of Radiation Oncology at UNC who was on her own journey to discover life after cancer. I attended several of Carolyn's workshops and one about food, exercise and mindfulness changed my life and my way of thinking. While time has passed and passions cool, the basic ideas and concepts I learned from Carolyn are still near to me today. I'm careful about what types of food I put into my body; I try to practice mindfulness and I am diligent about my exercise. No, I'm still not one who wakes up at 5 each morning to pound the pavement, but I've found ways to get exercise into my life. I've learned that unless I'm playing tennis, I'd better get my exercise early in the morning or it won't get done. I've found exercise buddies who walk with me or go to the fitness room with me and often, we end our sessions with a quick coffee before heading to work. I actually find that I miss it when I'm away from my regular exercise routines.

So now, I'm nearly seven years away from the initial diagnosis. My life has changed, but I'm so grateful for many of those changes. I try to remember "not to sweat the small stuff" and while exercise didn't turn me into a slim, blonde, thirty year old (I still struggle with my weight) probably the best change has been the steady course of exercise that I have folded into my life. I feel good afterwards and because I choose to exercise with various buddies, I get the added advantage of a good dose of friendship mixed in with the health benefits. As a close friend of mine said when we were playing a tennis match and we were down five games to two, little baby steps, that's all we need. We came back and won that set! So I say: take the chance, try it and you'll see that the little baby steps can be the key, it was for me.

Self-Assessment: Part II

How much do you exercise?

Take a look at your recreational physical activity for the past week. How often did you take a walk, and for how long? Did you play tennis? Swim? Practice yoga? Get on the treadmill? Bike? Your recollection doesn't have to be perfect, and you might want to use a typical week scenario. But be honest with yourself about what you usually do.

Note that we are talking about recreational physical activity, not everyday activity. While housekeeping or shopping or climbing the stairs at work does indeed provide physical activity, the studies that we have discussed specifically measured the amount of time and intensity of activities undertaken for exercise above and beyond the daily activities. If you do physically strenuous work, this may not apply to you.

This is exactly how they collect the data for the studies just reviewed. Fill out the first two columns on the form below to determine your baseline exercise level. You don't have to start on a Monday; pick whichever day of the week was yesterday and work your way back. Fill out the activity and time spent engaged in that activity columns.

Day	Activity	Time	Met	Met-hr
Monday				
Tuesday				
Wednesday				
Thursday				
Friday				
Saturday				
Sunday				

Here is how you fill in the last two columns. For each activity, look up its Met assignment on the *Compendium of Physical Activity Tracking Guide*, is found at: www.prevention.sph.sc.edu/tools/docs/documents_compe ndium.pdf.

Some common values are:
Moderate walking = 3
Light biking on a stationary bike = 3
Yoga = 3.5
Jogging = 7
Running = 8
Aerobic class = 8
General health club training = 5.5
Tennis = 7
Swimming breast stroke = 10

Insert the Met value in column four for each activity, and then multiply by the time (in fraction of hours) for column five.

Now that you've filled out your table for a typical week, add all of the values in the Met-hours column to determine your Met-hours per week average activity level.

We hope that your weekly total exceeds 9 Met-hours. If so, congratulations! Keep up the good work.

If you are not quite making it, take a look at this table. Do you want to reduce your risk of death by one third? Get at least 3 Met-hours/week of exercise. By half? Shoot for 9 Met-hours/week.

Reduction in Risk of Death

Study	3-9 Met-hr/wk	9+ Met-hr/wk	Increase after dx
NHS	31%	44%	
CWLS*	35%	41-56%	
HEAL*		50%	
WHI		46%	33%
WHEL	35%	50%	
ABCPP		27%	
* death due to breast cancer			

Self-Awareness: What helps you exercise?

We hope that you received a strong recommendation from your health care team to exercise when you'd finished treatment (or even during treatment - studies show that it is safe, and beneficial). Surprisingly, the vast majority of breast cancer survivors do not follow the exercise recommendations. In fact, some studies show that breast cancer survivors are actually more likely to decrease their levels of physical activity after diagnosis, by an average of two hours per week (1). Women who are heavier are more likely to do so.

Why is this so? Time, motivation, fear, depression, there are a host of reasons. But we suspect that one reason is that people don't know or understand how very effective exercise is at preventing breast cancer recurrence and death. It bears repeating: this is one of the most effective things you can do.

What are **your** barriers to exercise? What stands in the way of implementing and persisting with an exercise program that is right for you? Take a moment to list a few of the factors that you need to overcome to adopt healthy exercise habits.

<u>Five reasons why I don't exercise as much as I'd like to or should:</u>
1.
2.
3.
4.
5.

Now, look at it another way. Perhaps you do exercise regularly, or perhaps you did in the past. What are the conditions that help you to exercise?

<u>Five things that make it easier to exercise regularly:</u>
1.
2.
3.
4.
5.

Sometimes taking the time to analyze your motives and the factors that help or hinder you can be very illuminating. It is likely that for many people time is a barrier. If we look at the time it takes to carve 30 minutes out of our day to do something so good for us, most of us can find it somewhere. Perhaps one of the barriers is that exercise isn't enjoyable. In that case, find a physical activity that is. What are the factors that help you to exercise? Your dog, perhaps? One study shows that women who have a dog get more exercise from walking their dogs. Friends? A fun and energetic yoga group? Exercising with others is a great help; knowing that someone will be looking forward to exercising with you helps you to make sure that you do. How about trying something new? Embarking on a challenging Tai Chi course can get you out of a rut and look forward to doing something new each week. Do you already have a healthy exercise program? Perfect. Take a few minutes to remind yourself of the choices that you have made that enable you to continue to take care of yourself.

As you track your exercise over the next several weeks, develop a deeper awareness of what works and what doesn't work for **you.** When impediments or excuses arise, see them for what they are and think about how to work around them, or with them. Choose to put yourself in situations that favor an active lifestyle. Are you ready for that tennis club membership? Go for it!

Call to Action: Part II

This week's assignment is simple. Get at least 3 Met-hours of exercise this week. Better still, aim for nine. It doesn't matter what you do, so pick something that you enjoy. If you need suggestions, check out the Met website for activities. If you are short on time (aren't we all), perhaps you want to pick something with a higher MET level and do it for a shorter time. Make sure, however, that you pick something that is right for your level of conditioning. Remember, exercise during and after treatment is **safe**, but use common sense.

Track it. In the notebook that you started for your daily weight (you're still doing that, right?), add a note of the type and duration of exercise each day. At the end of the week (or daily, if you like), calculate the Met-hours as we did for the self-assessment.

Develop your awareness. As you do each exercise, note what you had to overcome to do it, and note what made it easier. Add to the list you started in the self-assessment to track the barriers and the aids to your exercise program.

By the end of the week, you will probably already be feeling better. Especially when you think about how you are doing your part to reduce your risk. Go back to the Table of Self-Assessment II and bask in the glow of the column which shows that you just pushed yourself into the drastically reduced risk of death group!

Finally, take a few minutes to explore the resources available to you in your community. At the University of North Carolina Cancer Hospital, we have a fantastic exercise program developed specifically for breast cancer survivors called "Get Real and HEEL." Many YMCA's and similar community programs have inexpensive or free exercise classes for cancer survivors, supported in part or fully by the Lance Armstrong Foundation. Cancer center support programs can be a great resource to identify exercise groups that provide both the social and physical benefits of cancer recovery programs. UNC's Cancer Support Program has a vibrant yoga community, as does Cornucopia House, a private support center. These programs offer a supportive way to embark on a life-long exercise program, and to try something new in a risk-free way. If you are self-motivated, an excellent resource is The Breast Cancer Survivor's Fitness Plan from Harvard Medical School, written by Carolyn Kaelin. We urge you to explore your options, and try something new whenever your exercise regimen is getting too ho-hum.

References: Part II

1) Ballard-Barbash R, Friedenreich C, Courneya K et al. Physical activity, biomarkers, and disease outcomes in cancer survivors: a systematic review. J Natl Cancer Inst 2012; 104:815-40.

2) Chlebowksi R. Nutrition and physical activity influence on breast cancer incidence and outcome. The Breast 2013; 22:530-37.

3) Bianchini F, Kaaks R, Vainio H. Weight control and physical activity in cancer prevention. Obes Rev 2002; 3:5-8.

4) Holmes M, Chen W, Fiskanich D et al. Physical activity and survival after breast cancer diagnosis. JAMA 2005; 293:2479-86)

5) Ainsworth B, Haskell W, Leon A, et al. Compendium of physical activities: classification of energy costs of human physical activities. Med Sci Sports Exerc 1993; 25:71-80.

6) Holick C, Newcomb P, Trentham-Dietz A et al. Physical Activity and survival after diagnosis of invasive breast cancer. Cancer Epidemiol Biomarkers Prev 2008; 17:379-86

7) Irwin M, Smith A, McTiernan A. Influence of Pre- and Postdiagnosis physical activity on mortality in breast cancer survivors: the Health, Eating, Activity, and Lifestyle Study. J Clin Oncol 2008; 26:3958-64.

8) Irwin M, McTiernan A, Manson J et al. Physical activity and survival in postmenopausal women with breast cancer: results from the Women's Health Initiative. Cancer Prev Res 2011; 4:522-9.

9) Bertram L, Stefanick M, Squib N et al. Physical activity, additional breast cancer events, and mortality among early-state breast cancer survivors: findings from the WHEL study. Cancer Causes Control 2011; 22:427-35.

10) Irwin M, Smith A, McTiernan A. Influence of Pre- and Postdiagnosis physical activity on mortality in breast cancer survivors: the Health, Eating, Activity, and Lifestyle Study. J Clin Oncol 2008; 26:3958-64.

11) Beasley J, Kwan M, Chen W et al. Meeting the physical activity guidelines and survival after breast cancer: findings from the after breast cancer pooling project. Br Cancer Res Treat 2012; 131:637-643.

12) Ibrahim EM, Al-Homaidh A. Physical activity and survival after breast cancer diagnosis: a meta-analysis of published studies. Med Oncol 2011; 28:753-65.

13) McTiernan A, Tworoger S, Ullrich C et al. Effect of exercise on serum estrogens in postmenopausal women: a 12-month randomized clinical trial. Cancer Res 2004; 64:2923-28.

14) Goodwin P, Ennis M, Pritchard K et al. Fasting insulin and outcome in early-stage breast cancer; results of a prospective cohort study. J Clin Oncol 2002; 20:42-51.

15) Pasanisi P, Berrino F, DePetris M et al. Metabolic syndrome as a prognostic factor for breast cancer recurrences. Int J Cancer 2006; 119:236-8.

16) Irwin M, Varma K, Alvarez-Reeves M et al. Randomized controlled trial of aerobic exercise on insulin and insulin-like growth factors in breast cancer survivors: the Yale Exercise and Survivorship study. Cancer Epidemiol Biomarkers Prev 2009; 18:306-13.

17) McTiernan A, Ulrich C, Slate S et al. Physical activity and cancer etiology: associations and mechanisms. Cancer Cases Control 1998: 9:487-509.

18) Chlebowki R, Aiello E, McTiernan A. Weight loss in breast cancer patient management. J Clin Oncol 20:1128-43, 2002.

19) Fairey AS, Courneya KS, et al. Effects of exercise training on fasting insulin, insulin resistance, insulin-like growth factors, and IGF binding proteins in postmenopausal breast cancer survivors. a randomized controlled trial. Cancer Epidemiol. Biomarkers, Prevent 2003; 12: 721-727.

20) Fauret AS, Courneya KS, Field CJ et al. Effect of exercise training of C-reactive protein in postmenopausal breast cancer survivors: A randomized controlled trial. Brain, Behav., and Immunity 2005; 19:381-388.

21) Fairey AS, Courneya KS et al. Randomized controlled trial of exercise training and blood immune function in postmenopausal breast cancer survivors. J. Appl. Physiol. 2005; 98: 1534-40.

22) Irwin ML, McTiernan A, Bernstein L et al. Physical activity levels among breast cancer survivors. Med Sci Sports Exerc 1994; 36:1484-91.

23) Courneya KS, Segal RJ, Mackey JR et al. Effects of aerobic and resistance exercise in breast cancer patients receiving adjuvant chemotherapy: a multi-center randomized controlled trial. J Clin Oncol. 2007; 25:4396-4404.

Part III: Diet Quality

Did you know that women who ate a high-quality diet after their diagnosis of breast cancer have a lower risk of death?

Did you know that eating seven servings of fruit and vegetables per day is associated with better survival?

Did you know that combining exercise with good eating is much more powerful than either alone?

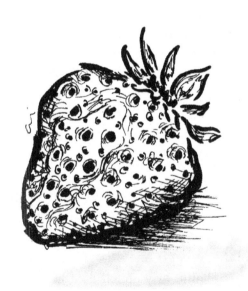

Diet quality

We've discussed weight control and exercise as two separate topics, but naturally they are intertwined. Women who exercise more tend to gain less weight. The converse can also be said: women who are overweight tend to get less exercise.

A similar situation exists for eating habits, or diet. A better diet is associated with better weight control. A better diet is also associated with getting more exercise. So, although we understand that in the real world we won't parse out how we eat from weight control, it might be of value to ask whether what we eat matters from a breast cancer recurrence standpoint, or whether all the benefit can be supplied by a diet pill or a gym membership.

One of the most common questions breast cancer survivors ask is, "What should I eat?" Does following a vegetarian, a Paleo, a macrobiotic, a Mediterranean, an Asian, an Ayurvedic, or a Western diet make a difference in breast cancer outcomes?

The effect of what we eat on any given outcome is an enormously complicated matter to figure out. We know that we all metabolize food in different ways. We also know that foods interact with one another, and with the effects on our bodies. Think of yourself as a living chemistry lab. The foods that you eat are like a variety of chemicals being poured into a test tube. The conditions of the reaction vary from person to person. Are you a quick metabolizer? Does your body's complicated p450 enzyme system handle the chemicals in turkey, for example, the same way that another person's body does?

Dietary factors are the subject of many different views because they are so complicated. Making clear recommendations is difficult because there is relatively little conclusive data. Initially, efforts focused on individual food components - vegetables, fats, carbohydrates, for instance. This is akin to asking whether aerobic exercise affects breast cancer outcomes, instead of asking whether exercise in general affects outcomes. More recently, studies have begun to generalize the dietary questions from single-focus to types of diets. This reflects an increasing appreciation of the way that different components of diet interact with one another in a *synergistic* way (where the two together are greater than the sum of the two combined), or even an *antagonistic* way (acting in opposing ways). Looking at overall diet quality attempts to take into account the complexity of the individual component interactions.

Our approach is to discuss the big picture first. We will look at "good" diets vs "bad" diets to see whether there is any difference between the two. If so, we will then turn our attention to whether we can dissect out specific components of the "good" or "bad" diets that are driving most of the effect.

It will be many years before we gain clear answer to whether, say, blueberries actually reduce breast cancer recurrence risk. In fact, it is doubtful that the clinical trials to give us that answer will ever be performed. In the meanwhile, we can use a "preponderance of evidence" approach. If there is an indication in the breast cancer population that a particular diet is helpful, and then if we can determine biological reasons for why certain food components may be active against breast cancer from the laboratory studies (which we will delve into in Part IV), and, most importantly, if the dietary recommendations are not harmful or even unpleasant, then we suggest that you consider it, in some cases strongly. Diet is a moving target, and we encourage you to take what you learn here and apply it to your own dietary choices.

The answer from a data standpoint can be simplified, however. Eat a "good" diet. Probably, most of us carry around a conviction that eating well is better than eating poorly. Does eating well really make a difference in breast cancer outcomes? The answer is, yes. Let's look at the studies.

Defining a good vs bad diet

Before we delve into the data, let's clarify just what, exactly, is meant by a "good" diet as opposed to a "bad" diet. It is important to understand how the studies are categorizing a wide array of eating habits in such as way that they can be grouped as "good" or "bad. It won't come as a surprise that there is not a uniform way of categorizing diets; different studies use different criteria. However, if we look at the variations, we can clearly see a consensus of how we can evaluate our own eating habits to determine which group we fall in.

There are four different diet scoring systems that are used in the studies that we will discuss in the next sections. They are similar in that they separate out healthy foods from junk food. Processed meats and chips are bad in every scoring system. Fruits and veggies, whole grains, and nuts are good in every scoring system. You probably already know intuitively which foods are healthy and which are junk, but if you want more detail, the following will give you specifics.

The Healthy Eating Index-2005 (HEI-2005) is a measure of diet quality that was created by the U.S. Department of Agriculture and the National Cancer Institute to assess conformance to U.S. Federal dietary guidelines for Americans in 2005 (1). "Good" components are: fruit, vegetables, grains, meat and beans, and oils. "Bad" components include saturated fats, sodium, solid fats, alcoholic beverages, and added sugars. This was revised to become the AHEI-2010, primarily by taking into account nuts and alcohol. The overall HEI score is the sum of 10 dietary components, weighted equally. Each component of the index has a maximum score of 10 and a minimum score of zero. The maximum overall HEI score is 100. Higher scores are better.

The HEI-2005 is actually pretty complicated to calculate, because it is normalized to the amount of calories. Furthermore, the amounts should reflect only the constituent and not the total amount of the foods in which they may be contained. For example, the fruit juice fraction of a juice drink, which may be only 10% of the total product, counts toward total fruit, but the rest of the beverage counts toward added sugars. Likewise, the skim milk fraction of whole milk counts toward the dairy constituent, but the butterfat in whole milk counts toward calories from solid fat. Determining the amounts of each dietary constituent contained in the total quantity of foods under consideration requires linking to relevant databases, as information on both nutrients and food groups are needed to calculate HEI scores. However, you can take a stab at calculating your own HEI-2005 score in Assessment III. It's a worthwhile, if somewhat painstaking, effort.

The Alternate Mediterranean Diet Scale (aMED) is similar in many ways to the HEI scores in that it encourages fruit, vegetables, legumes, whole grains, and mono-unsaturated fats. The aMED differs in that it does not penalize for modest alcohol use, but does for red and processed meats (the AHEI-2010 also emphasizes avoiding red and processed meats, but the HEI-2005 does not). The aMED also doesn't penalize for salt use, in contrast to the HEI scoring.

Another diet quality scoring system classifies diets as "prudent" vs "Western". The Western diet is one that includes high intake of meat, refined grains, and high-fat foods and dairy products. It has been associated with increased risk of coronary heart disease, stroke, diabetes, and colon cancer. In contrast, the "prudent" diet is characterized by eating more vegetables, fruits, fish, whole grains, nuts, low-fat dairy and legumes. The more Western-type foods consumed, the higher the Western diet score. The more the prudent foods consumed, the higher the prudent score. The data is then grouped into 4 categories of low to high Western diet and, separately, 4 categories of low to high prudent diet. While it is likely that those with a prudent style of eating are less likely to be classified as high Western style and vice versa, each score is analyzed separately in the data that we will discuss.

The most important concept for an individual breast cancer survivor to understand is the difference between a generally good versus generally bad diet. However, the fact that so many different measurements have been used in research studies makes it more difficult to draw comparative conclusions or to perform some of the meta-analysis type studies that gave so much credence to the results in the previous topics. The next several years should see a burgeoning consensus in this field, and thus offer us more robust conclusions. In the meantime, there is probably little practical difference in the definition of "good" vs "bad" amongst the different studies, so we will focus our attention on the results of each of the studies as if the distinctions are equivalent.

♀ Key Study: NHS

One of the earliest, large studies to ask about diet and breast cancer survival comes from the Nurses' Health Study (NHS) (2). We've discussed the NHS in Part I as it related to weight, and Part II as the study looked at exercise. The investigators next turned their attention to the question of whether how one ate was associated with outcomes in breast cancer survivors. As you may recall, the NHS was a large, population-based data collection study of over 120,000 female nurses. Of this larger group, 2,600 developed breast cancer over the course of the study, between 1982 and 1998, and had completed a dietary habits questionnaire.

The investigators classified the diets into two major patterns. The "Western" pattern was characterized by high intake of refined grains, processed and red meats, desserts, high-fat dairy products, and French fries. On the other hand, the "prudent" diet was characterized by fruits and vegetables, whole grains, legumes, poultry, and fish. Each woman's questionnaire data was scored as being higher or lower on the "prudent" scale and higher or lower on the

"Western" scale. So, in effect, there were two things to compare: high or low within each diet, and more prudent vs more Western.

Naturally, the investigators looked at a number of factors related to diet. The first was whether eating habits before diagnosis were associated with outcomes. They found that women who had a higher intake of the Western diet had a slightly higher risk of death from any causes, but that this was not statistically significant. Eating a prudent diet before diagnosis was not associated with any outcomes. Thus, diet **before** diagnosis didn't seem to have much impact on outcomes.

In contrast, diet **after** diagnosis did matter. Women who continued the Western style of eating after diagnosis were less likely to survive. In fact, they had a 47% higher risk of dying than those who least followed the Western diet. However, the difference in survival was not due to breast cancer. It was due to death from other causes than breast cancer.

The converse was also true. Women who most followed the "prudent" eating patterns were also **less** likely to die from causes other than breast cancer, 46% less likely than those who least followed a "prudent" diet.

♀ Key Study: LACE

The Life After Cancer Epidemiology (LACE) Study provides further evidence. The LACE study was an observational study of the lifestyle habits of early stage postmenopausal women recruited primarily from the Kaiser Permanente Northern California Cancer Registry (3). For 1,900 breast cancer survivors, food frequency questionnaires were used to classify scales of "prudent" vs "Western" diets. The participants were enrolled in the study within three years, but an average of two years after diagnosis. Women who developed a recurrence, or died early after diagnosis, were not included in the study, so this study relates primarily to later phases of survivorship and longer-term eating habits after diagnosis.

Diet was assessed using the Fred Hutchinson Cancer Research Center Food questionnaire, a self-administered semi-quantitative food frequency questionnaire with 122 food and beverage items. Food items were classified into 38 food groups based on nutrient profiles. Two distinct dietary patterns were identified: the prudent diet included more vegetables, fruits, fish, whole grains, poultry, nuts, and low-fat dairy. The Western diet was characterized by more consumption of red meat, processed foods, fried potatoes, sweets, and, interestingly Italian and Mexican foods.

The investigators found that the women who were in the top quarter of eating a prudent diet had 43% lower risk of death over the roughly six years of follow up in the study than those who were in the lowest quarter of eating prudent-diet containing foods. Conversely, women who were the highest partakers of a Western diet had a more than 50% higher risk of death compared to those whose diets were least characterized by Western-style eating habits. As with the NHS, the differences in survival between healthy and non-healthy eaters were not in the risk of breast cancer deaths, but in deaths from other causes.

It bears repeating that the risk of death in these early stage breast cancer survivors was nearly as high from other causes of death as it was for breast cancer. Of the women who died of non-breast cancer causes in this study, 30% died of cardiovascular disease, 17% from other cancers. Due to the design of the study, which focused on better prognosis breast cancers and excluded those who developed recurrence within the first two years of diagnosis, the risk of breast cancer recurrence in this study was very low. Thus, an effect of diet on breast cancer recurrence would not be expected to be very large compared to an effect on other causes of death.

It is also important to note that diet parallels other health behaviors that we know are important. Higher prudent pattern scores were seen in women who were also more physically active, and had gained less weight from year one before diagnosis to enrollment. Higher Western pattern scores were seen in women who were younger, heavier, had gained more weight, and had smoked at some point in their lives.

The LACE study confirmed the results of the NHS. Both studies showed similar improvements in overall survival, but not breast cancer survival, with a more prudent diet. Indeed, the results were strikingly similar, despite the differences in follow-up time (the NHS had 20 years of follow-up compared to the LACE 6 years). Both studies showed similar improvements in survival with a prudent diet, and both had nearly identical rates of death due to cardiac disease.

♀ Key Study: WHI

The Women's Health Initiative Study (WHI) recruited more than 160,000 postmenopausal women from 40 clinics to participate in an observational and clinical trial study that looked at health behaviors. Of the larger group, 2,317 women developed breast cancer and had filled out a dietary questionnaire after their breast cancer diagnosis. The survey asked which of 122 component items they ate, how often, and how much. This data was then scored using the HEI-2005. Participants were then followed over time to see whether there were differences in survival between groups with different diet quality scores.

Over an average time period of follow-up of almost 10 years, the investigators discerned a difference in survival in groups of women with different HEI-2005 dietary scores (4). Women who ate a higher quality diet (top quarter) had a 26% lower risk of death from any cause than women who ate less well (bottom quarter of the scoring). Again, the difference wasn't due to breast cancer. The investigators found that a better quality diet significantly reduced (by 42%) the risk of dying from causes other than breast cancer. Since the average 10-year survival for women diagnosed with early stage breast cancer is now about 90%, a near-halving of the risk of death from other causes is highly relevant.

In fact, most of the deaths that occurred were not related to breast cancer, but mostly due to cardiovascular disease or other cancers. There is ample evidence to support the relationship between a healthy diet and reducing the risk of cardiovascular disease, so the reduction in risk of non-breast cancer deaths is not surprising. Nor was it a shock to find that the women who ate a better diet were also more likely to exercise, to consume fewer calories, and to have a lower BMI.

The investigators of the WHI study published a follow-up to this study to look at the relationship between diet quality and survival in the larger cohort of women in their study, not only those who developed breast cancer. For this more recent study, they evaluated diets using four different diet quality indices: the HEI-2005, the HEI-2010 (or adjusted HEI, AHEI-2010), the Alternate Mediterranean Diet Score (aMED), and the Dietary Approaches to Stop Hypertention (DASH). This study confirmed their earlier findings of a significant relationship between better quality diet and improved survival; women consuming better quality food had an 18-26% lower risk of death due to any cause, or death due to cardiac disease or cancer (5). Furthermore, the results were strikingly similar regardless of which diet quality measurement was used. If you are reading this as a healthcare professional, take note – this applies to you too.

♀ *Key Study: HEAL*

We discussed The Health, Eating, Activity, and Lifestyle (HEAL) in Part II as it pertained to exercise, but the investigators of this study also looked at diet quality. As you may recall, this was a study to collect data on nearly 1,200 women diagnosed with breast cancer to study the relationship between lifestyle factors and breast cancer outcomes. In addition to the questions about exercise practices, the investigators asked about eating habits. Six hundred and seventy women from the study filled out detailed food frequency questionnaires that the investigators then used to score according to the Healthy Eating Index-2005 scoring system (6).

The HEAL study confirmed the WHI study findings; a better quality diet is associated with a reduced risk of death. In the HEAL dataset, the impact was even greater; those in the top quartile of diet quality had a 60% lower risk of death than those in the lowest quarter.

The HEAL study also showed something that the other studies had not. Better diet quality was also associated with improved breast cancer survival. **Women who had the best diet quality were 88% less likely to die from breast cancer than those with the lowest diet quality**.

While the HEAL study results agree with the WHI results, the magnitude of the benefit is much greater in the HEAL study. Why? No one knows for sure, but here are a few differences between the studies to ponder.

The HEAL study was specifically looking at dietary habits 30 months after diagnosis, since the investigators were interested in the long-term effects of diet on breast cancer outcomes. This means that anyone who suffered a breast cancer recurrence before this time-point would not be included in the study. It also implies that diet over time may be more relevant to the risk of death after breast cancer. If you improve your diet now, you may see the benefits years down the road.

Second, the HEAL study included both premenopausal and postmenopausal women, while the WHI study strictly looked at postmenopausal women. Third, the HEAL study represents a more diverse population, including more African American and Hispanic women because of their recruitment tactics (using databases to target regions with different social demographics).

It is worth noting, however, that the number of participants in the HEAL study was smaller than the WHI study. This results in greater statistical uncertainty. In other words, the magnitude of the benefit in the HEAL study may not really be all that different than the WHI study because the range of the possible actual benefit is greater, anywhere from 98 to 1 percent by the time one takes into account all of the factors of the multivariate analysis.

Health behavior controlled clinical trials

Although population studies can draw associations between behaviors and outcomes, only randomized controlled trials can address causation. The studies we've just discussed show a relationship between good eating habits and improved survival, but they do not prove that survival was better because of the good eating habits. There are other behaviors associated with good diet, such as better exercise habits and weight control that could just as well account for the better outcomes.

The only way to prove whether diet improves outcomes is to identify a group of breast cancer survivors up front, and then randomly divide them into two groups: those who are directed to follow a particular diet, and those who are not. Then one can compare the difference between the two groups. If there is a difference, we can be confident that the difference was due to the diet.

Randomized controlled trials work well to test the efficacy of treatments, like chemotherapy regimens or radiation therapy. However, it is much more difficult to be sure that a randomized trial of a health behavior like diet is truly measuring what you think it is measuring. After all, everyone eats. We haven't yet designed or implemented the diet trial that controls everything that people eat. An additional uncertainty is that the health behavior randomized trials usually rely on participants to vouch that they followed the prescribed diet. It's not like chemotherapy or radiation therapy, where a health professional administered a specific dose of a specific agent. Health behavior studies are much more fuzzy.

Nonetheless, at least two randomized controlled trials looked at diet and outcomes in breast cancer survivors.

♀ Key Study: WINS

The first large-scale randomized controlled clinical trial to test whether a dietary intervention could improve breast cancer recurrence was the Women's Intervention Nutrition (WINS) Study (7). The study asked whether a very low-fat diet would be achievable by breast cancer survivors, and, if so, whether this would reduce the risk of recurrence or of a second breast cancer.

Between 1994 and 2001, more than 2,400 women were randomized to receive intensive dietary counseling to follow a low-fat diet (the intervention group), or standard counseling to support healthy eating habits (the control group). The target for the intervention group was to get breast cancer survivors to consume 20% or less of their calories from fat, which was a reduction of roughly one third of the usual fat intake.

The women in the intervention succeeded in meeting their goals, which is, in itself, a major achievement of the study. Dietary change is difficult, but breast cancer survivors prove again and again that we are capable of doing so. Even the control group improved their fat intake somewhat, but not nearly as much as the intervention group.

However, the study investigators were unable to meet their goals. The study terminated prematurely due to discontinuation of the grant that was funding the research. This is a travesty that occurs all too often in lifestyle intervention studies. In the current fiscal climate, it is incredibly difficult to get funding to start such a study, let alone finish it. We need to raise our voices to demand that studies that do not have big pharma to fund and champion them still get a place at the table, even if they will make no company a profit. They still have the potential to save countless lives, to prevent many women from suffering a breast cancer recurrence.

That is exactly what the investigators did find from this study, regardless of not being able to carry it out as far as they wished; the low-fat diet prevented breast cancer recurrence and development of second breast cancers. When the study was terminated prior to the date that they had planned to assess the outcomes (3 years after enrollment of the last participant), the investigators evaluated the data anyway, even though early. They found that the women randomized to the low-fat diet group had a **24% reduction in the risk of breast cancer recurrence** compared to the control group. In absolute numbers, this translates into 3.6% reduction in breast cancer events. In other words, the results of this study predict that 3-4 out of every 100 breast cancers survivors would be less likely to develop a recurrence of breast cancer in the first 5 years after treatment on the basis of following a low-fat diet alone.

Let's say that we all agree that a 3.6% absolute benefit from something that costs next to nothing and has no nasty side effects is a no-brainer for a recommendation to implement such an intervention across the board. This is, after all, a randomized, controlled clinical trial. Why do we still question whether a low-fat diet is indicated for all breast cancer survivors? Because there is debate as to whether the benefit seen in this study was due to fat restriction.

One of the most interesting findings from the WINS trial is that women in the low-fat diet group lost weight, while women in the control group did not. It wasn't a lot of weight, but it was a few pounds, and it was statistically significant. You will recall from Part I that there is a strong link between weight maintenance and breast cancer recurrence, so many people have asked whether the positive results from this trial were due to the weight loss or due to the low-fat diet. Would another healthy diet give the same benefit as a low-fat diet?

We don't have the answer to that yet. Not surprisingly, given the awesome complexity of our bodies, it's not likely to be a simple answer. In the meantime, this study provides firm evidence that reducing fats to a target of 20% of calories is an excellent weight-control approach for breast cancer survivors, is not harmful, and has been as well-proven as possible to reduce the risk of developing breast cancer recurrence or a new breast cancer.

Good vs bad fats - the CWLS

It has become clear that the "fats" question is far more complicated than a "low-fat" vs "high fat" question. Not all fats are created equal. Not all are bad. In fact, some dietary fat (or, more precisely, fatty acids) are downright good. We are only beginning to scratch the surface on the complicated underpinnings of the way our bodies use fat just as we are only beginning to gain a better foundation on the variability of carbohydrate sources. Let's look at some of the underlying themes, from a breast cancer survivor standpoint.

First, it is pretty clear that one of the divisions between "good" fats and "bad" fats can be the distinction between saturated or trans fats and unsaturated fats. Saturated fats are fatty acids that have more hydroxyl groups along their chain, more branching points, and can generally be thought of as more stiff, less fluid. Think of a grove of brambly trees with lots of branching close to the ground vs a grove of tall bamboo where you can easily slip through the bases even while the breeze causes the entire grove to sway. Unsaturated fats are typically liquid and slippery; saturated fats are firm and sticky. Trans fats are artificially created by bombarding saturated fats to make even more branching. They have a longer shelf life in the grocery stores, and have become ubiquitous in the unhealthy "Western" diet.

All well in theory, but does it really make a difference for breast cancer survivors? The investigators of the Collaborative Women's Longevity Study (CWLS) asked that question. The CWLS was a study of nearly 4,500 breast cancer survivors who provided information via questionnaire on their lifestyle habits. Noting that the WINS trial (as well as the WHEL trial that we've discussed in Parts I and II) both contained a low-fat dietary intervention that made no distinction between "good" fats and "bad" fats, the investigators of the CWLS tapped their database to determine whether specific types of fat sources were associated with outcomes (10).

They used a 126-item food frequency questionnaire that asked number of servings of meat, dairy, fruit, and vegetable intake per day. Meat and dairy were further grouped based on their fat content. Meat was then examined separately based on type, whether poultry, fish, beef, or processed. Slightly less than half of the women queried were within 5 years of diagnosis of breast cancer, the rest were further out; therefore, this is a single point-in-time query of post-treatment eating habits.

The investigators found that total fat intake was not associated with breast cancer survival, or survival overall. However, the type of fat intake was. Women who were in the upper fifth of trans fat intake had a **78% increased risk of death** from any cause compared to those in the lowest fifth. Similarly, women with a median intake of 13% of total calories from saturated fat had a 41% increased risk of death from any cause compared to women consuming a median of 7% of calories from saturated fat. These findings support the hypothesis that type of fat matters - at least for survival. There were no significant differences in breast cancer outcomes.

It may be worth noting that this study provides a snapshot of American eating habits. Women in the lowest fifth of fat intake still consumed 23% of their calories from fat, while those in the highest fifth gained almost 40% of their energy intake from fats. Recall that the WINS trial successfully brought fat intake down to 20% in their intervention group.

Dairy fats

The CWLS study found that meat and dairy were two of the largest contributors to saturated fat. Dairy fat (to be more specific, U.S. style dairy fat) is also a major contributor of estrogenic hormones. Current mega-agro practices involve the milking of pregnant cows, who have high levels of circulating hormones. To add insult to injury, from an estrogen standpoint, the cows are also fed modified feed that promotes more hormone production. Thus, the question arises: is the harm from saturated fat ingestion observed by the CWLS investigators due to milk fat?

Investigators of the Life After Cancer Epidemiology (LACE) study directly addressed the question of whether high vs low dairy fat intake would be associated with breast cancer outcomes, hypothesizing that if the estrogenic hormones in American dietary fat were a factor, women who consumed more high fat dairy would fare worse (11). Similar to the CWLS study, the LACE study recruited women who had been diagnosed with breast cancer to fill out food frequency questionnaires. This study, however, added one more step. They queried women both at baseline (sometime after diagnosis) and then again 5 years later.

The investigators saw no association between overall dairy intake and outcomes. They did, however, find that high fat dairy intake was associated with worse survival, including increased risk of death from breast cancer. However, just as the CWLS investigators had found, the high fat dairy intake went hand in hand with trans-fat intake. Thus, it is difficult to determine which is the culprit.

This point is underscored by the findings of a similar study performed in Italy. The Italian study likewise did not find a difference in outcome between breast cancer survivors who consumed more dairy than those who consumed less. However, in contrast to the LACE study, they also saw no indication of any association between high fat dairy consumption and worse outcomes, for either breast cancer or survival (12).

As the investigators of the two studies point out in their back-and-forth debate, there are two major differences between the consumption of dairy in the two studies. In the American study, the majority of high-fat dairy was in the form of butter. Italians rarely use butter; they use olive oil instead. Olive oil has been shown to have significant health benefits, and, as we will discuss, may tip the balance of fats in a favorable direction. Second, there are significant differences in the farming practices between Italy and America. American milk may be unhealthier due to the manner in which it is produced. Indeed, the investigators of the LACE study state, "we would expect that associations between high-fat or low-fat dairy and breast cancer survival might differ depending on a country's predominant farming practices" (13).

What's the bottom line? By all means, go ahead and drink your milk. But choose wisely. If you can buy wholesomely produced milk, that may be better for you. If not, skim milk may be a wiser choice. Either way, remember that the data thus far shows a benefit for consuming less than 20% of your calories from fat. Unless, that is, you can keep your weight within optimum range with the amount of fat that you do regularly consume.

Biology: A balanced approach

Fat biology is complex. Our bodies need fat to function, but, as you are no doubt aware, too much fat is bad. But is it too much fat? Too much cholesterol? Too high a low density lipoprotein profile, or too low a high-density lipid profile? We can't even gain consensus on how metabolic endpoints of fats should look chemically in our blood. It's mind-boggling.

The omega chain fatty acids can illustrate some important points, from the breast cancer standpoint. Omega chain fatty acids are essential fatty acids that differ in the position of their side chains. Those that have a side chain in the 3rd position are called omega-3 fatty acids. Those with a chain in the 6th are omega-6, those in the 9th position are the omega-9 fatty acids.

It seems like a small distinction in an otherwise large and sophisticated molecule. But consider this for a moment: omega-6 fatty acids have been shown to stimulate breast cancer cell growth in laboratory studies, while omega-3 fatty acids inhibit breast cancer cell growth. Omega-6 fatty acids are important in inflammation, which also sets up an environment favorable to breast cancer proliferation.

These opposing effects are further amplified by the complex interplay between the two molecules in our bodies. The higher the omega-6 intake, the lower the omega-3 levels because of feedback inhibition loops that affect the processing of omega-3 fatty acids. And the reverse appears also to be true. There is a seesaw effect between the two. Furthermore, other fatty dietary factors, such as certain polyphenols found in Mediterranean diet components can increase the levels of omega-3.

So the relevant question would be: do levels of omega-6 and omega-3, or the balance of the two, affect outcomes for breast cancer survivors? We don't yet have that answer, but we do have data on omega-3 and omega-6 fatty acid intake and risk of breast cancer. An evaluation of 21 studies performed through 2012 showed that intake of marine omega-3 polyunsaturated fatty acids was associated with a reduced risk of developing breast cancer (8). For every 100 mg increase per day, the risk of developing breast cancer was reduced by 5%. In another compelling study, Danish investigators measured levels of marine omega-3 fatty acids in the breast tissue of women with breast cancer and women without breast cancer who were undergoing breast reduction procedures. The investigators found higher levels of marine omega-3 fatty acids in the tissue of the women without breast cancer compared to those who developed breast cancer.

Thus, there appears to be a rationale for increasing omega-3 fatty acids and reducing omega-6 fatty acid intake to prevent breast cancer development, which as we've discussed is still relevant for those who still have breasts. However, to date there is no data to indicate whether there is a benefit to improving the omega-3: omega-6 balance to prevent breast cancer recurrence. We will likely see this eventually, given the favorable effects on inflammation from an omega-3 favored balance. Furthermore, there is every indication that this will also be favorable from a cardiac standpoint.

There is one study of omega-3 and omega-6 fatty acid intake in breast cancer survivors that brings up another intriguing reason for breast cancer survivors to boost their omega-3 intake. It may significantly improve post-treatment fatigue. Fatigue is one of the most common and debilitating complications of breast cancer treatment. While we know relatively little about the causes, and importantly, treatments of fatigue, studies suggest that fatigue among cancer survivors may be driven by altered cytokines and stress hormones that contribute to a high inflammatory state. This can be affected by diet. We will delve more deeply into this issue in Part IV.

♀ Key Study: WHEL

Now that we've discussed fats in detail, let's add fruits and vegetables to the mix. The Women's Healthy Eating and Living (WHEL) trial was designed to ask whether a diet very high in vegetables, fruit, and fiber but low in fat reduced the risk of breast cancer recurrence, development of a second breast cancer, or death (14). The study investigators randomized slightly more than 3,000 women who had finished treatment for early stage breast cancer to follow a very high fruit/vegetable and low-fat diet versus following the standard guidelines of 5 or more servings of fruits and vegetables per day. The roughly 1,500 women who had been assigned to the intervention group (diet group) participated in a telephone counseling program, cooking classes, and newsletters. All participants were periodically asked to report what they had eaten the previous 24 hours.

The investigators took steps to verify that participant's reports of following the prescribed diet were accurate. Blood was collected at certain points to determine whether markers of fruit and vegetable consumption showed that the intervention group was consuming more fruits and vegetables than the control group. Lipid profiles were checked to determine whether the low-fat diet group was consuming less fat. As hoped, the investigators confirmed that the women in the intervention group did, indeed, report eating more servings of fruits and vegetables than the control group. Furthermore, they ate less fat. The blood studies confirmed the reports from participants about what they were eating, in that they showed that women in the intervention group had higher levels of carotenoids and better lipid profiles than those in the control group.

Despite high fruits and vegetables and low-fat diet, the intervention group did not have any improvement in breast cancer recurrence/new primary or in survival. The two groups were nearly identical.

This well-performed randomized trial has been widely quoted as showing that diet has no effect on outcomes in breast cancer survivors. That may, indeed, be true. However, there are some important caveats to consider before generalizing that conclusion.

First, this study does not disagree with the findings of the other studies of diet quality we've already discussed, because this was not a trial of "good" vs "bad" diet. It was a study of "good" vs "better" diet. Why do we say that? Because the control group in this study already met the criteria of the high quality or prudent diet of the other studies. At the time of enrollment, participants in both groups already consumed an average of 7 servings per day of fruits and vegetables. This increased by 65% for vegetables and 25% for fruits in the diet group, but it also increased slightly for the control group. Thus, one conclusion that can be drawn from this study is that eating 12 servings of fruits and vegetables per day does not improve outcomes over eating 7 servings per day of veggie/fruit diet. In other words, this study proves that "better" is not superior to "good", not that "good" and "bad" diets are equivalent. There was no low quality diet arm on this study.

Along the same theme, that this is a "better" vs "good" diet study, we find that very few women died of causes other than breast cancer. Recall that cardiac deaths accounted for nearly half of the deaths in the "good" vs "bad" diet studies. In this study, only seven cardiac deaths occurred in the entire 3,000-strong group. This certainly supports the idea that 7 servings of fruits/veggies per day is beneficial from a cardiac standpoint, with apparently little to gain from more.

Another indication that the control group's "good" diet is good enough is that neither the control group nor the intervention "better" diet group gained weight over the 7-year course of the study. This is further evidence that even the control group in this study is already on the right track.

Thus, far from concluding that "diet doesn't matter", one can conclude that this study supports the concept that eating well does matter. We can also conclude that "better" is not superior to "good". While this study proved that women can, and will, stick to very strict diets, there is a great deal of comfort to be gained to know that we don't necessarily have to. If you are following good eating habits, going all the way to a more extreme diet may well be going overboard.

The CWLS data found that typical American breast cancer survivors consumed far fewer servings of fruits and vegetables than recommended. Only the top quarter got on average 5 servings in per day, while the lowest quarter had just over one. Contrast this to the WHEL group, where the top half ate 5 or more servings per day. It may not be surprising that the CWLS study found no benefit from eating more fruits and vegetables. "More" in this case may hardly be adequate.

The WHEL investigators addressed this issue. If one conclusion from their study is that "better" doesn't add, could they relook at the data to gain a sense of how "good" is good enough? At least in terms of fruit and vegetable servings? They asked this question by looking at the control group, the group that we called the good diet group. Yes, the control group followed a good diet on average, with seven or more servings of fruits and vegetables. But if this group was divided the middle, the median number of fruits and vegetable servings was right around five. The investigators divided them into four even groups based on quartiles of fruit/veggies consumption, and asked whether there was a difference in outcome between these groups of more modest fruit and vegetable consumption.

And there was. Survival significantly improved with increasing intake of vegetables and fruits to 5 or more servings per day (15). Breast cancer survivors who consumed more than 7 servings of fruits and vegetables per day had only an 8.3% risk of death. Women who fell into the lowest quartile of fruits and vegetable consumption, less than about 3 1/2 servings per day on average, had the highest rate of death, a 12.4% risk of death over the course of the study.   This is a difference of four women out of 100 who are alive at the end of the study in the seven or more fruit and veggie group compared to those who eat fewer than 3 1/2 servings. This is huge!

⚕ *Key Study: Hormone-diet interactions*

As you are probably well aware, different breast cancer types respond to different treatment approaches. For example, estrogen and progesterone receptor expressing breast cancers respond to endocrine treatments such as tamoxifen or aromatase inhibitors while estrogen receptor negative breast cancers do not. Is the same true for dietary interventions? Are some types of breast cancer more susceptible than others? Who might benefit the most from dietary interventions?

We might expect that hormone receptor negative breast cancers would benefit more from the beneficial effects of a good diet, at least in the short run. One reason for this is that hormone receptor negative breast cancers are less effectively treated by medical therapies, and more likely to recur. Thus, there is more to be gained from any improvement. Conversely, hormone receptor expressing breast cancers are treated with endocrine therapy that lasts for a long time, typically five years. The effects last even longer, so it would take a long time to see the influence of diet above and beyond this treatment. Since the WINS study results were analyzed at an early time-point (less than five years), we would expect that women with hormone receptor expressing tumors would still be receiving effective endocrine treatment. Diet may not add much to that in the short term.

One of the benefits of well-conducted clinical trials is that they can continue to provide a treasure-trove of high-quality information long after the main endpoints of the trial have been met. There is a robust database of carefully defined and selected parameters just sitting there, waiting to be mined. Although secondary analyses have to be taken with a grain of salt because they aren't the *a priori* defined primary endpoints, they can shed a great deal of light on a wide range of additional questions.

With this in mind, the investigators of the WINS study asked whether there was a difference in the benefit of a high-quality diet depending on hormone receptor status of the tumors. As they hypothesized, the low-fat diet appeared to have a greater effect on preventing relapse in women with estrogen receptor negative tumors (7). Breast cancer survivors who had estrogen or progesterone receptor negative tumors who were in the diet arm of the study had 42% lower risk of recurrence than those in the control arm, while those with receptor positive tumors had only a 15% reduction in the risk of recurrence or death. These results were not conclusive, however, as they were not certain (they did not reach statistical significance).

The WHEL study investigators used the data from their study to investigate further the question of hormone receptor-diet interactions that the WINS study suggested. You may recall that there were relatively few cardiac or breast cancer-related deaths in this study, probably reflecting that the study population was already, on the whole, pretty healthy. But what if one looks at a subpopulation that has a worse breast cancer prognosis in this group? Perhaps a subset that might be expected to benefit from better diet? That's exactly what the study investigators did.

Studies have shown that both a low-fat diet and increased fiber can lead to 20-25% lower levels of circulating estrogens (16). The WHEL study investigators hypothesized that the low-fat, high vegetable (and high fiber) diet in their study would provide more benefit to those women who had higher circulating estradiol and worse prognosis. How might you select out these particular women? You could pick those who did not develop hot flashes after treatment, because those are likely the ones who have higher levels of circulating estrogens.

That's what the WHEL investigators did (17). From the parent study, they had nearly 3,000 women for whom they had collected information on hot flashes. The 900 who did not have hot flashes were evenly divided between those who were randomly assigned to the "better" diet and the "good" diet. It appeared that the WHEL investigators could ask their secondary question. So what did they find?

They found a significantly lower rate of breast cancer recurrences in the women without hot flashes who followed the low-fat, high fruits and vegetable diet compared with those who did not. For this particular subset of women, the risk of recurrence was about a third less in the group who followed the "better" diet than the "good" diet. These results suggest that diet is exerting at least some of its beneficial effect through mitigation of hormone stimulation of breast cancer cells. This effect on hormones may be masked in the short term by endocrine therapy, which has a much stronger effect on hormone responsiveness of breast cancer cells. But it may be increasingly important over time, and for endocrine therapy unresponsive tumors.

Does this mean that you should pay particular attention to reducing fat and increasing fiber if you did not develop hot flashes after treatment? Possibly. However, there are some caveats to such "secondary analyses". Since the trial wasn't specifically designed to test this question, one cannot conclude that the trial "proves" that this is the case. However, it does point a finger clearly in that direction. It would take another trial that specifically selected up-front those women who had not developed hot flashes and then randomized them to the intervention or control groups. Unfortunately, to our knowledge, no such trial has yet been designed.

So what to do in the meanwhile? This secondary study suggests that a "better" diet is not superior to a "good" diet, except possibly for those women with higher circulating levels of hormones, i.e. those who did not develop hot flashes after treatment. You know who you are; you can decide whether the data is compelling enough to increase the fruits and veggies to 12 servings per day, and the fat down to 20% of your caloric intake. For the rest of us, there may be some consolation to those pesky hot flashes. We can eat an ice cream once in a while, or, better yet, use olive oil freely. A nice, creamy hummus, anyone?

♀ Key Study: Diet plus exercise WHEL & HEAL analysis

While we are on the subject of "knock-on" studies, or subset secondary analyses of larger, randomized studies, there are more pearls that we can glean from the Women's Healthy Eating and Living Study (WHEL). (As an aside, aren't you glad that these investigators kept plugging away at the data, even long after the original endpoints had been met? This is another advantage to providing a healthy budget for clinical trials. When investigators have to scramble, often unsuccessfully, to get together the pittance of funding to perform the analysis of these value-added studies, it leaves so much untapped, so much wastage. We can raise our voices to change that. After all, it's our data too).

The WHEL investigators looked at other factors that we've seen to be relevant from other studies. As others have shown, they found that being heavier at the time of diagnosis was associated with worse overall survival. Also, exercising more was associated with better survival. None of these findings should surprise us. But then the investigators did an interesting thing. Recognizing that many of these factors are inter-related, for instance, those who eat better tend to exercise more and to be less heavy, they asked whether the combination of exercise and diet had more of an effect than either alone.

What they found was striking. Women who fell into the top half of veggie/fruit consumption and the top half of exercise had much better survival (18). In fact, they had *half the risk of death* as those who were less active and ate fewer veggies and fruits, or even those who did only one or the other. Indeed, women in this study who were physically active and ate a modest amount of fruits and vegetables had a 10-year survival of 93% as opposed to 86% for those who were not active and did not eat the minimum of fruits and vegetables. **This absolute survival benefit of 7% is higher than the benefit achieved by almost every advance in breast cancer treatment, to put it in perspective.** Furthermore, the benefit was just as great for those women who were heavy, and who were at increased risk of dying.

How much did they have to exercise? How many veggies and fruits? How extreme the lifestyle? Not much. All it took to be in the clearly best group was to eat 5 or more servings of fruits and vegetables per day, and to exercise more than 9 Met-hors/week. That should sound familiar; it's the same conclusion we reached from the exercise studies discussed in Part II.

Note the power of the combination of the two factors, diet and exercise. This is evidence to support what is suspected; a combination of good habits is even more potent than adding them together. The combination is *synergistic*; the effect of the two together is far greater than simply adding the individual effects. Exercise benefits the effects of diet, and diet benefits the effects of exercise. They interact in a powerful way.

It is important that a secondary analysis such as this one be validated. The WHEL secondary study was put to the test with an independent (unrelated) dataset. In yet another example of the benefits that can be derived from a well-created and well-maintained dataset, the HEAL investigators were able to look to their study to see whether they, too, would see a greater effect from combining both good diet and exercise.

The results were spectacular (19). Compared with inactive survivors with poor-quality diets, active survivors with better quality diets had an **89% reduced risk** of death from any cause and a **91% reduced risk** of death from breast cancer. Although this is not a randomized, controlled trial, and thus doesn't afford the highest level of proof, with these numbers it would be highly unlikely that the benefit is not real. In short, while exercise is good, and a healthy diet is good, the combination is extremely good medicine.

♀ Key Study: Diet and fatigue

We've been discussing the impact of diet quality on survival, but there are other important quality of life factors that are improved by a healthy diet. Simply put, eating well makes you feel better. Let's look at one well-performed study that illustrates the point.

The most frequent, distressing, and under treated cancer symptom reported by cancer survivors is fatigue (20). We will discuss fatigue and its biologic underpinnings in greater detail later, but let's take a peek at fatigue as it relates to our subject at hand. The investigators of the HEAL study asked whether diet quality was associated with fatigue (21). AHEI-2010 scores and physical activity were calculated from 770 breast cancer survivors in the HEAL study who had completed diet and physical activity surveys at 30 months after diagnosis. Patients were evaluated roughly between three and four years after diagnosis.

Women with better quality diets had significantly less fatigue than those who ate poor quality diets. Women who had higher quality diets also tended to be older, exercised more, consumed fewer calories, and had lower BMIs than those who ate a poorer quality diet. However, even counting out these imbalances between the groups, breast cancer survivors who had the highest quality diet had lower total fatigue, as well as lower fatigue in each of the areas measured. In other words, although exercise, body habits, and other health habits may play a role, diet quality alone did improve fatigue even if not considering the improvements from these other factors.

When the investigators looked at the data further, they found that one component of diet drove the majority of the effect; empty calories (soda, chips, etc.) were associated with significantly more fatigue. There are very few things that have been shown to ameliorate fatigue after breast cancer. **Avoiding empty calories** is one of those. Isn't it nice to know that you have to power to improve your energy level?

The investigators of this study parsed out a complicated relationship between fatigue, diet, and exercise. While both exercise and diet improved fatigue, the strongest effect of diet on fatigue was seen in those who got some exercise, but not as much as recommended. This intuitively makes sense. For those who are getting plenty of exercise, the negative effects of the empty calories may not be very relevant. After all, if you just ran 5K, who cares about a bag of potato chips afterward? However, if you aren't getting quite enough exercise, that bag of potato chips may have a much more deleterious effect. Finally, if you are a total couch potato and get no exercise, even a high quality diet isn't going to make up for it. It could work the other way as well. If you feel too tired to get even a little exercise, a good diet alone isn't going to be enough to bring you up the way a bit of exercise can.

♥ Key Study: Diet and quality of life

It seems intuitive that eating well would make you feel well. There is one study that looked specifically to see whether this is truly the case, asking whether diet quality, as measured by the Diet Quality Index, was associated with measurements of either physical or mental quality of life. Seven hundred and fourteen breast cancer survivors who participated in the HEAL study (and hadn't had a recurrence) reported their dietary habits, and then, 10 months later, several quality of life factors (22).

Breast cancer survivors who ate a higher quality diet scored significantly better on three out of four mental health quality of life scores and two of four physical quality of life scores. Women who ate better were more likely to perform normal social activities without interference due to physical or emotional problems than those who ate a poor diet (47.4 vs 44.9%). They were more likely to experience no problems with work or other daily activities as a result of emotional problems (41.9 vs 36.1%). They also felt more peaceful, happy, and calm (51.5 vs 47.8%). From a physical standpoint, women who ate a higher quality diet were better able to perform physical activities without limitations due to health (45.5 vs 42.4%), and more likely to have no pain or limitations due to pain (52.7 vs 48.9%).

This study is an epidemiological study, so doesn't establish cause and effect. It is possible that diet reflects a better quality of life, not that it leads to it. However, other studies have specifically addressed whether improved diet leads to improved quality of life in non-breast cancer populations and found that changing diet for the better did, indeed, lead to improved quality of life. Further supporting the findings of the HEAL study, a smaller study also found an association between better diet quality and two measures of quality of life, depressive and menopausal symptoms (23).

It is likely that many more studies will follow, as this is an important point. If eating better can improve quality of life, this is one more powerful tool that breast cancer survivors can use to aid their recovery to a happy, healthy life. Eat well!

Prescription: Part III

Eat well

The evidence:

- Nurses' Health Study (NHS) found that breast cancer survivors whose diet most typified a Western diet had a 47% higher risk of death than those who least followed a Western diet. Conversely, those who followed a prudent diet were 46% less likely to die than those whose diet was less prudent. The difference in death rates was due to causes other than breast cancer, primarily cardiac and second malignancies.

- The Life after Cancer Epidemiology (LACE) Study found that breast cancer survivors who followed a Western diet had 50% higher risk of death, while those who followed a prudent diet had 43% lower risk of death.

- The Women's Health Initiative Study (WHI) found a 42% reduced risk of death for breast cancer survivors who were in the top quartile of diet quality as opposed to those in the lowest.

- The Health, Eating, Activity and Lifestyle Study (HEAL) found an 88% reduced risk of breast cancer death for those who ate the highest quality diet compared to lowest. This study population differs from the above studies, including premenopausal breast cancer survivors and more African American and Hispanic women. It also looked at longer-term effects of diet, excluding those who had recurred or died within the first two years of diagnosis.

- The Women's Interventional Nutrition study (WINS) *randomized controlled trial* found that women randomized to a very low-fat diet had 24% lower risk of breast cancer recurrence compared to the control group. Despite early termination of the study, a 3.6% absolute reduction in breast cancer events was demonstrated.

- The Women's Healthy Eating and Living (WHEL) study randomized breast cancer survivors to a diet very high in fruits, vegetables, and fiber and low in fat vs usual diet. No difference in breast cancer events or survival was seen. Breast cancer survivors in the intervention arm ate an average of 12 servings of fruits and vegetables per day, compared to 7 in the control arm. Events were extremely low, consistent with the healthy diet in both arms.

- WHEL secondary analyses looked at whether more fruit and vegetable consumption had any effect. They found an absolute survival benefit of 4% when comparing groups that consumed less than 3.4 servings of fruits/vegetables per day compared to more than 7, death rates of 12.4% vs 8.3% over the course of the study.

- Secondary analyses from the WINS and WHEL studies suggest that a low-fat, high fiber diet is most beneficial for breast cancer survivors with ER/PR negative tumors, or those with higher levels of circulating estrogens as evidenced by lack of hot flashes.

- Diet and exercise together yield strongly beneficial results. The WHEL study demonstrated an absolute 10-year survival benefit of 7% in those who consumed 5 or more servings of fruits/vegetables per day in combination with 9 Met-hours per week of exercise. The HEAL study confirmed and expanded this secondary analysis, finding that breast cancer survivors who were active and ate high quality diets had an 89% risk reduction in death from any cause and 91% reduced risk of death from breast cancer compared to inactive survivors with poor-quality diets.

- A high quality diet is associated with reduced fatigue, particularly in those who get less than the recommended amount of exercise. The strongest correlation with fatigue was the amount of empty calories consumed.
- A high quality diet is associated with improved mental and physical quality of life, including parameters of social functioning, emotional and role functioning, mental health, physical functioning, and bodily pain.

Lisa's eating well story

Like many women, I have struggled with my love of food and my weight for my entire adult life. Weight Watchers has been my "go to" for success to lose weight; however, I lost weight by often using my "daily points" on unhealthy fast foods I craved. My breast cancer diagnosis (Stage 1 ER positive) was my wake-up call to take care of my health, not just my weight.

As fortune or fate would have it, I learned of the New Life *after* Cancer "Prescription for Healthy Behaviors" Lecture and Cooking Classes a year after my breast cancer diagnosis and treatment. Dr. Carolyn Sartor's lectures with facts and insight on what mattered with regard to eating resonated: maintain a healthy weight, avoid insulin spikes, important as I already had insulin resistance due to PCOS and a family history of diabetes, and eat lots of fruits and vegetables.

For the past four years, I have since built on these principles and evolved my cooking and eating to make healthy and delicious versions of my favorite foods which are heavily plant based and extremely low in added sugar and refined flour. I have lost 40 pounds, normalized my high blood sugar and borderline high cholesterol, and celebrated five years without a breast cancer recurrence!

Here's how I did it:
First, I educated myself on healthy eating by reading lots of books on the Mediterranean Diet which has been well studied for its impact on health; as well as other favorites including Dr. Andrew Weil's *Anti-Inflammatory Pyramid*,

Dr. Joel Fuhrman's *The End of Dieting,* and Dan Buettner's *The Blue Zones.*

Secondly, I educated myself to improve my cooking skills. I use Cooks Illustrated's *The Science of Cooking* and Cooks Illustrated online to which I refer frequently to learn the techniques to prepare whole foods to make them taste delicious.

Thirdly, I educated myself on batch cooking and storage to simplify cooking and to eat with minimal preparation during the week. I prepare large batches of proteins, grains, and vegetables once or twice a week and refrigerate them or freeze them in portion size glass containers. Thus I only have to defrost in microwave and/or do minimal cooking for each meal.

I also decided this year to see a registered dietician to help me pull it all together, which has accelerated my healthy habits change and my weight loss. My dietician helped me outline an eating plan to help regulate my blood sugar and eliminate, **yes eliminate**, my food cravings! I discovered it was not just **what** I ate but **how** I ate which made a world of difference.

As a footnote, I allow myself an occasional indulgence. My weekly treat is a chocolate croissant! I moderate its impact on my blood sugar, which I learned from Carolyn, by eating it after a high fiber bowl of steel cut oats with blueberries and walnuts.

Self-Assessment: Part III

How good is your diet?

Now it's your turn to see how your diet rates. Let's take a stab first at the HEI-2010. This system is fairly cumbersome. In fact, there is a free statistical macro that you can use to calculate your HEI score (see www.cnpp.usda.bov/healthyeatingindex for more information). You can also look up full details at: http://www.cnpp.usda.gov/sites/default/files/healthy_eatin g_index/HEI2010-UpdatePaper.pdf. Oh, and if you don't make it all the way through this exercise, be sure to skip to the end of this assessment to do it the easy way.

We can do an abridged calculation by making some approximations, however. Start by writing down everything you ate or drank yesterday, including amounts. That's a bit tough, right? Do you remember everything? Do you remember it accurately? You can probably already see one of the main criticisms of this type of research - the dependence on accurate recall and reporting. That's OK, just do your best. Or, if you feel better about it, do a typical day. It doesn't have to be perfect, but it should be honest about your usual eating habits.

Next, look at your list of foods. Did you eat any fruit? Give yourself 5 points if you ate more than 0.8 cups per 1,000 calories. Aha! You see the next difficulty. In order to accurately calculate the points, you need to know how many calories you consumed over the course of the day because each of the amounts of food type are defined as a portion of a 1,000 calorie load. This makes sense, since someone who eats twice as much as another doesn't necessarily have a better diet unless they eat twice as much fruit to go with the extra calories. However, it makes it difficult to calculate your actual HEI-2010 unless you have all of the data.

Food	Score
Total fruit	
Whole fruit	
Total vegetables	
Greens and beans	
Whole grains	
Refined grains	
Dairy	
Total protein	
Seafood and plant	
Fats	
Sodium	
Empty calories	

If you want an accurate representation, **a nutritionist can help you through this**. Otherwise, let's continue with the quick and dirty. Give yourself a score of 5 (best) to 0 (worst) for eating fruit. If you ate more than 1.5 servings you get a 5. If you ate none, you get a 0. If you ate somewhere in-between, give yourself an intermediate score. Next, do the same for eating a whole fruit, not a component of fruit. Score 5 if you ate more than 2 1/2 cup servings. What is the difference between whole fruit and fruit? Mainly juice. Next, give yourself 5 points if you ate more than 2 cups (4 servings) of vegetables, less if you ate less, o if none. Finally, give yourself extra points if you had dark green vegetables, beans, or peas, 5 points for 1 serving or more.

Next, let's move on to whole grains. Give yourself 10 points for eating more than 3 ounces, less for lesser quantities, and o for none. Now, the reverse side of grains. Did you consume refined grains yesterday (flour, bread, white rice)? If less than 3 ounces, give yourself a 10. If more than 8 ounces, give yourself a o. If in-between, guess an appropriate score, remembering that you get more points for consuming less refined grains.

How about dairy (milk, yogurt, cheese, and soy beverages)? Give yourself 10 points for more than 2.5 cups and dial it down to o points for none. For protein, give yourself a 5 if you had more than 5 ounces, o for none, or somewhere in between. A separate category is used for seafood and plant protein (nuts, soy, etc). Give yourself 5 points if you had more than 1.5 ounces, o for none. You may have noticed that this gets a bit tricky. Do you count beans as protein or vegetables? It depends on how much protein you're getting. If you need the beans to get enough protein, count it first in protein. Put the extra into vegetables. But don't count twice.

Moving on to fats. This, too, gets tricky to calculate because the score relates to the ratio of poly- and monounsaturated fatty acids to saturated fatty acids. In other words, you need to know the types of fats in your food. The technical definition for a score of 10 is if the polyunsaturated and monounsaturated fats are more than 2.5-fold the saturated fats. The definition of a o is if they are less than 1.2-fold. Let's make it simple. If your fats came mostly from nuts and olive oil, give yourself a 10. If they came mostly from processed foods and chips and desserts and red meat, give yourself a 0.

Finally, two more components that we want to minimize: sodium and empty calories. If you had more than 4 grams of sodium, give yourself a 0. If you had less than 2, give yourself a 10. If you got more than 50% of your calories from empty calories, defined as calories from solid fats, alcoholic beverages, and added sugars or other junk food, give yourself a 0. If you had less than 20% of your calories from those sources, give yourself a 10.

You did it! Congratulations for wading through this. It **is** painstaking, even with the simplifications. Don't worry, we will get on to easier scoring systems next, but this should at least help you to understand how the data from the WHI study was scored. Now, the moment you've been waiting for: add up your scores to see your approximate HEI-2010.

My HEI-2010 score = _____

Now that you have an approximate score, where do you fit in the WHI results?

If your score is above 77: Congratulations! You are in the group with a 26% reduced risk of death compared to those whose score is less than 63.

If your score is 71-77: You are in the group with a 14% reduced risk of death.

If your score is 63-71: You are in the group with a 7% reduced risk of death.

If your score is below 63: You are in the highest risk group.

How do the HEAL study results apply to you?

If your score is above 74: You are in the group with a 60% reduced risk of death **and** an 88% reduced risk of death from breast cancer.

Going through this exercise can help you to see how little you may need to change your diet to fall into a better prognosis group. The slope between 63 and 77 is pretty steep, and as you've just experienced from scoring your diet, a few more servings of fruits and vegetables, or whole grains instead of refined can make a big difference in your score.

To make it **much more simple**, ask yourself two questions:

How many servings of fruits/vegetables do I eat per day?

How much exercise do I get per week? (You've been keeping your exercise log from Part II, right? And getting more than 9 Met-hours per week?)

If you consume more than 5 servings of fruits and vegetables per day **and** exercise at least 9 Met-hours per week, CONGRATULATIONS!!!! By doing so, you have **halved** your risk of dying in the next 10 years, according to the WHEL study. According to the HEAL study, you have reduced your risk of dying from breast cancer by 91%!

Not quite there yet? Let these figures motivate you!

Self-Awareness: What do you like to eat?

Often, our eating choices have more to do with what's convenient, easy, or habit. Following a specific diet can be quite difficult, not only to maintain, but also to set up so that you can quickly grab a bite that conforms to the diet.

But what if we make it easier? What if it's a choice between taking the nuts from the vending machine as opposed to the chips? We've just seen that choosing items associated with a prudent diet as opposed to a Western diet is associated with significantly improved survival. Can it really be that simple? Actually, yes.

Below is a list of the "prudent" vs "Western" foods. Take a good look at it. Are there foods that you like on the prudent side as much or almost as much as the Western? Why don't you reach into the refrigerator for a broccoli snack today instead of a piece of bread? It may be that you don't have a ready-made broccoli snack on hand. You can change that easily enough.

Circle your favorites on the prudent list. Cross off the items on the Western list that you don't necessarily care for. Think about how you can choose to change from butter to olive oil, from refined baked goods to whole wheat baked goods. When you shop, start adding a few more prudent foods to your list while you simultaneously avoid buying some of the Western foods.

Change begins with awareness. Study this list carefully. Notice that the items in each list are ranked in order by the weight they are given in scoring each diet. In other words, eating cruciferous vegetables gets you the highest rating on the prudent scale, while eating cold cereals, while not bad, doesn't count as much in your favor. Conversely, eating red meat is considered most typical of a Western diet, while eating eggs is still Western, but not weighted as adversely. So as you look at each list, factor in the impact of your decisions. Do you want a sweet? That's not so bad, in moderation. It's pretty low on the list of foods to avoid. Your entrée choice has more of an impact than having a dessert in moderation, especially if it's a vegetarian entrée. Become aware of the quality of your diet, and making good choices will follow. Especially when you consider that it really does make a big difference, not only in survival, but also in how you feel.

Foods in the Prudent Diet	Foods in the Western Diet
Cruciferous vegetables	Red meat
Other vegetables	Processed meats
Tomatoes	Creamy soups/sauces
Dark yellow vegetables	Butter
Fruits	Mayonnaise
Legumes	Americanized Italian foods
Onions	Fried potatoes
Leafy vegetables	High-fat dairy
Fish	Fried chicken
Soups	Snacks
Whole grains	Refined grains
Poultry, not fried	Pasta or potato salads
Salad dressings (all)	Mexican foods
Rice, grains, plain pasta	Sweets
Fruit juice	High-energy drinks
Low-fat dairy	Eggs
Nuts	Organ meats
Potatoes, not fried	Cold cereals

Call to Action: Part III

Like last week's assignment, this week's assignment is straightforward. Eat at least 5 servings of fruits and vegetables per day if you exercise, 7 if you don't. And, keep up with your exercise, and keep weighing in.

Track it. In your notebook, record the number of servings of fruits and vegetables each day, along with your exercise and your weight. We hope that you are noting a trend toward the better as the weeks unfold. Did you make your goal of 9 Met-hours per week last week? When you add the veggies this week, you will benefit from the synergistic combination of the two. And the added bonus of seeing these good habits reflected in your weight.

Develop your awareness. As you make choices in what you eat this week, how many times do you comfortably exchange an item from the Western diet for one from the prudent diet? Stock your fridge and workplace with your favorites from the quality diet list. Be mindful of what you eat. Under what circumstances to you choose to eat something less healthy? Do you really want to, or is it a default action or reaction? What can you do to tip the balance toward the healthy choices?

By the end of the week, you will probably already be feeling better. How is your energy? Your strength? If you like, take a few minutes to redo the self-assessment crude calculation of your HEI score. Did it improve? Have you bumped up to one of the more favorable categories?

Finally, take a few minutes to explore the resources available to you to support healthy eating habits. One option is to try out a cooking class that promotes healthy eating, such as New Life *after* Cancer's Food for Thought workshop. Another option is to try out a food delivery service like Blue Apron or Hello Fresh. Through a subscription, you can bypass meal planning and grocery shopping to receive weekly deliveries for fresh, healthy meals that you cook, following the provided recipes. The quality of the meals is excellent, and the preparation reasonably straight-forward. It combats the default of eating out too often when you don't want to go through the hassle of meal planning and shopping, or preparing something that isn't as well-balanced or rewarding. What are the resources that will help you to eat more healthfully? Avail yourself of them!

References: Part III

1) Guenther PM, Reedy J, Krebs-Smith SM. Development of the Healthy Eating Index-2005. J Am Dietetic Assn 2008; 108:1896-1901.

2) Kroenke C, Fung T, Hu F et al. Dietary patterns and survival after breast cancer diagnosis. J Clin Oncol 2005; 23:9295-9303.

3) Kwan M, Weltzien E, Kushi L et al. Dietary patterns and breast cancer recurrence and survival among women with early-stage breast cancer. J Clin Oncol 2009; 27:919-26.

4) George S, Ballard-Barbash R, Shikany J et al. Better Post-diagnosis diet quality is associated with reduced risk of death among postmenopausal women with invasive breast cancer in the Women's Health Initiative. Cancer Epidemiol Biomarkers Prev 2014; 23:575-83.

5) George SM, Ballard-Barbash R, Manson JE et al. Comparing indices of diet quality with chronic disease mortality risk in postmenopausal when in the Women's Health Initiative Observational Study: Evidence to inform national dietary guidance. Am J of epidemiology 2014; 180:616-25.

6) George S, Irwin M, Smith A et al. Post diagnosis diet quality, the combination of diet quality and recreational physical activity, and prognosis after early-stage breast cancer. Cancer Causes Control 2011; 22:589-98.

7) Chlebowski R, Blackburn G, Thomson C et al. Dietary fat reduction and breast cancer outcome: interim efficacy results from the Women's Intervention Nutrition study. J National Cancer Inst 2006; 98:1767-76.

8) Zheng J, Hu X, Zao Y et al. Intake of fish and marine omega-3 polyunsaturated fatty acids and risk of breast cancer: meta-analysis of data from 21 independent prospective cohort studies. BMJ 2013; 346:3706-76.

9) Alfano C, Imayama I, Neuhouser J et al. Fatigue, inflammation, and omega-3 and omega-6 fatty acid intake among breast cancer survivors. J Clin Oncol 2012: 30:1280-87.

10) Beasley J, Newcomb P, Trentham-Dietz A et al. Post-diagnosis dietary factors and survival after invasive breast cancer. Breast Cancer Res Treat 2011; 128:229-36.

11) Kroenke C, Kwan M, Sweeney C et al. High and low fat dairy intake, recurrence, and mortality after breast cancer diagnosis. J Natl Cancer Inst 2013; 105:616-23.

12) Zucchetto A, Francheschi S, Polesel J et al. Re: High- and low-fat dairy intake, recurrence, and mortality after breast cancer diagnosis. J. Natl Cancer Inst 2013: 105: 1759-60.

13) Kroenke C and Caan B. Response to Zucchetto et al. J Nat Cancer Inst 2013; 105:1761-2.

14) Pierce J, Natarajan L, Caan B et al. Influence of a diet very high in vegetables, fruit, and fiber and low in fat on prognosis following treatment for breast cancer: the Women's Healthy Eating and Living (WHEL) randomized trial. JAMA 2007; 298:289-98.

15) Pierce J, Stefanick M, Flatt S et al. Greater survival after breast cancer in physically active women with high vegetable-fruit intake regardless of obesity. J Clin Oncol 2007; 25:2345-51.

16) Wu A, Pike M, Stram D. Meta-analysis: dietary fat intake, serum estrogen levels, and the risk of breast cancer. J Natl Cancer Inst 1999; 91:529-34.

17) Gold E, Pierce J, Natarajan L et al. Dietary pattern influences breast cancer prognosis in women without hot flashes: The Women's Healthy Eating and Living Trial. J Clin Oncol 2008; 27:352-59.

18) Pierce J, Stefanick M, Flatt S et al. Greater survival after breast cancer in physically active women with high vegetable-fruit intake regardless of obesity. J Clin Oncol 2007; 25:2345-51.

19) George S, Irwin M, Smith A et al. Postdiagnosis diet quality, the combination of diet quality and recreational physical activity, and prognosis after early-stage breast cancer. Cancer Causes Control 2011; 22:589-98.

20) Curt G, Breitbart W, Cella D et al. Impact of cancer-related fatigue on the lives of patients: new findings from the Fatigue Coalition. Oncologist 2000; 5:353-60.

21) George S, Alfano C, Neuhaouser M et al. Better post diagnosis diet quality is associated with less cancer-related fatigue in breast cancer survivors. J Cancer Surviv 2014; 8: 680-87.

22) Wayne S, Baumgartner K, Baumgartner R et al. Diet quality is directly associated with quality of life in breast cancer survivors. Br Cancer Res and Treat 2006; 227-232.

23) Tangney C, Young J, Murtaugh M et al. Self-reported dietary habits, overall dietary quality and symptomatology of breast cancer survivors: a cross-sectional examination. Br Cancer Res and Treat 2002; 71:113-123.

Part IV: How Do Diet and Exercise Work? The Biology behind Inflammation

Did you know that inflammation is linked to worse outcomes after breast cancer?

Did you know that exercise and healthy eating practices not only reduce inflammation but also improve immune function and reduce tumor growth factors?

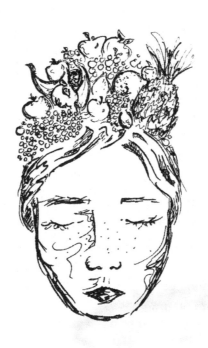

The party analogy for tumor growth

We've talked about how shifting the balance between omega-6 and omega-3 polyunsaturated fatty acids affects inflammation, but a side trip into tumor biology might be in order to put this into perspective and raise awareness as to how health behaviors affect several biological processes involved in tumor growth, and even improve treatment side effects.

Tumor growth factors, growth factor receptors, inflammation, and immunity are key players in cancer progression and response to treatment. To better understand the biology, we offer an analogy. Imagine a teenager who is left home alone on a Friday night while his parents attend a fundraiser. Like the cells in our bodies, he is a well-intentioned teenager, but there are many influences at work that might pull him off the track of the straight and narrow and into a path that can lead to increasing levels of chaos and destruction. In our analogy, his home represents a normal cell, the doors of his home represent normal cell growth factor receptors, and friends represent growth factors.

One Friday night, a friend stops by. He happens to bring along a six pack of beer. He is invited into the house and steps in through the front door. As the two sit down to watch the game on TV while they drink the beer, they are like your normal cell that has just been fed by a toxin. It's not that big a deal, unless . . .

Three beers each later, they decide it's a good idea to call another friend who might have more beer. Sure enough, he is ready and available, and comes over with another six pack. By now, they are primed to gulp that down pretty quickly and start thinking about who else they can invite over. By now, it's becoming a party. Judgment has taken a back seat, and, although they know that what they are doing is wrong, they don't really care anymore, already disinhibited under the influence of the beer.

"Disinhibited" is a very good description of what happens to a normal cell when it first becomes a cancer cell. Technically, we call it "deregulated", meaning that it has lost its normal regulatory control to not grow, not replicate (divide), not invade surrounding tissues. In our analogy, the first step along this path was the beer, and for our cells, sometimes the first step is imbibing a *growth factor* that the cell normally shouldn't be getting, or not getting too much of.

The growth factors that are most relevant to breast cancer cells are some that you will readily recognize: estradiol (estrogen), epidermal growth factor (EGF), insulin and insulin-like growth factor. Too much of these, handled the wrong way, in a cell that doesn't say "no" can initiate cancer, or in our analogy, can initiate the party. It's a pivotal step from a normal cell to tumor cell. This is why diet and exercise, by reducing levels of these growth factors, inhibits the growth of tumor cells.

But three teenage boys drinking two six packs of beer are a much smaller problem than what can happen next. When they run out of beer again, they call another friend. Good news from the party's perspective, bad news from the perspective of a happy, healthy evening. The friend they call is already at another party, and it's hopping. They are already primed, and they surge *en masse* to the boy's house.

There are hundreds of them, and lots and lots of beer. And they just can't seem to all get in and out of the door at the same time, which is what they want to do, to get to the fridge to eat all of the food. So, they knock out a window, or two, and start creating more entrances.

The growth factor *receptors* on the cell surface are like the doors of the house. The growth factors bind to the receptors, and in doing so, activate signaling that instructs the cascades to initiate growth, genetic effects, and production of new growth factors. Breaking down the windows and creating more doors is like amplifying HER2, a very important receptor for breast cancer cell growth. Women with HER2 positive cancers have tumor cells that have learned to make many, many, many doors, that is, many HER2 receptors. This makes them much more sensitive to the growth factors that bind to HER2, or, in our analogy, beer toting teens going through doors and windows.

The epidermal growth factor receptor (EGFR) is another example of what can go awry at this stage. Breast cancer cells don't typically create a massive amount of extra EGFR, but they do readily make the ones that exist more efficient, in part by creating their own EGF. In our analogy, instead of breaking windows to create more entrances, the party gets organized, and they set up coolers outside in the yard to ensure that a plentiful supply of beer is readily at hand.

Another example relevant to breast cancer that this phase of the party analogy represents is the growth factor, insulin, and its relative insulin-like growth factor. You are probably already well aware that diet and exercise influence levels of insulin in your body. As growth factors, insulin is represented by the beer in our analogy. But, since these are particularly potent signaling molecules, let's say that they aren't beer, but something related like marijuana.

When either the supply of growth factors (tumor cells can make their own) or their availability to the cells is deregulated, we see *tumor progression*. The situation has definitely gotten out of hand, and it's going to take a lot more to clean it up at this point.

So, by this time, there are hordes of beer-drinking and marijuana-smoking teens permeating the house and spilling out all over the lawn. If this is a law-abiding, well patrolled neighborhood, by now someone would have called the cops. However, if this is a home in an area where partying is the norm, perhaps this activity wouldn't raise any eyebrows. Indeed, there may even be another party the next street over and the two will eventually fuel each other.

The interaction between neighborhood and the party house is similar to the interaction between our bodies and the tumor, called the *host-tumor interaction*. The host-tumor interaction is particularly important in the regrowth and spread of already treated tumors. One of the key players in the host-tumor interaction is our immune system. Our natural killer cells (NK cells) are white blood cells whose job it is to patrol the neighborhoods and nip problems in the bud. This is also called *immune surveillance*. When things get out of control, the NK cells are joined by a host of other inflammatory mediators to try to keep the lid on the party.

But, just as a scenario of cops breaking up a riot, things can get quite out of hand when you have a revved up tumor and a revved up inflammatory reaction. In our analogy, you can think of the inflammatory reaction as the neighborhood. A well-ordered, non-chaotic inflammatory background allows for a smooth-functioning immune reaction. A revved up, already brewing inflammatory background is more like the neighborhood that is used to partying and already has a few underway. The immune system doesn't stand much of a chance in that environment. In fact, the inflammation may make things worse.

From this analogy, you can see how growth factors such as insulin, growth factor receptors such as HER2, immune mediators such as NK killer cells, and inflammation all play a role in tumor progression and regrowth. All of the lifestyle factors that we discuss in this book impact one or more of these pathways.

♀ Key Study: Inflammation and survival

From the party analogy, you can appreciate how the baseline inflammatory state, the neighborhood in our analogy, can influence both the promotion and progression, but also the likelihood that the party will not ever get under control. Let's see whether that stands up in the reality of breast cancer. Does inflammation influence breast cancer control?

You may recall that the Health, Eating, Activity, and Lifestyle (HEAL) study was discussed in both the exercise and diet chapters, and also showed us the interaction between diet and exercise. Knowing that chronic inflammation is a key contributor to breast cancer progression, the investigators asked whether breast cancer survivors who have higher levels of inflammation were at increased risk of recurrence. The majority of the participants in the study had given blood samples to be used to assess the levels of the inflammatory markers C-reactive protein (CRP) and serum amyloid A (SAA). CRP and SAA are non-specific inflammatory proteins that are produced in response to some of the cytokines that we will discuss in further detail, interleukin-6 and tumor necrosis factor alpha. CRP doesn't tell us anything about the source of inflammation, but it is a reliable marker of inflammatory states. In terms of our analogy, it is a general gauge of the neighborhood, like the average number of calls to the Police Department per night. It doesn't tell us which houses the calls come from.

The HEAL investigators found a strong and highly significant relationship between elevated inflammatory markers and decreased survival in this cohort of over 700 breast cancer survivors (1). Women who were in the highest third of inflammatory marker levels (CRP > 3.9 mg/L) had 2.27 times the risk of death than those with the lowest levels of inflammatory markers (CRP less than 1.2 mg/L).

There was a correlation between breast cancer recurrence risk and inflammatory marker levels, but it wasn't quite as strong as the survival risk. This may, in part, be due to the design of the study. In order to remove the confounding effect of tumor cells on increasing the inflammatory response, they removed from the equation women who had already had evidence of recurrence. This would factor out some potentially strong associations between inflammation and recurrence. Nonetheless, there did still appear to be an association between chronic low-grade inflammation and breast cancer outcomes.

Interestingly, it appeared that there wasn't a dose-dependent increase in risk with higher levels of CRP. It appeared that if inflammation was above a certain level, the increased risk occurred. In terms of our analogy, once the neighborhood was permissive of out of control parties, it didn't matter if it became more so.

If inflammation is associated with worse survival and disease recurrence, we may perhaps improve outcomes by reducing inflammation. To find out how to combat inflammation, we can look first to see what factors are associated with higher levels of inflammation. Then, we can identify what to target.

The HEAL investigators asked which demographic, lifestyle, and clinical factors in their database were associated with higher concentrations of CRP (1). They found several factors.

First, concentrations of CRP and SAA were strongly linked. This makes sense, since both are inflammatory markers. However, they measure different processes and may be relevant to distinct outcomes. For example, levels of SAA do not correlate with fatigue, while CRP does (more later).

Higher age, smoking, BMI, and waist circumference all were strongly related to elevated levels of inflammatory markers. We can't do much about age, but we can change BMI and waist circumference through diet and exercise, as we've already discussed. Indeed, more physical activity was strongly associated with lower levels of inflammatory markers.

Let's look at more studies that investigate at the relationship between inflammation and exercise or diet.

🔑 Key Study: REHAB

Knowing that inflammation is associated with survival naturally leads to the important question: what can reduce inflammation? Exercise has been associated with lower levels of inflammatory markers in the general population, and may be one way to reduce inflammation in breast cancer survivors. Exercise is associated with reduced levels of inflammatory markers, but this doesn't prove that exercise actually reduces inflammation. To see whether this is the case, one would need a randomized trial of exercise vs no exercise to look at whether CRP levels differed between the two groups. A Canadian group did just that.

The Rehabilitation Exercise for Health after Breast Cancer (REHAB) study was a randomized, controlled trial that looked at effects of exercise in postmenopausal women who had breast cancer (2). Fifty-three breast cancer survivors were randomized to train on an exercise bicycle 3 times weekly for 15 weeks, or not. Levels of CRP were checked at the beginning and at the end of the 15 weeks.

Breast cancer survivors who exercised had a decrease in their CRP levels (average decrease of 1.39 mg/L), but women who were randomized to the control group did not (if anything, they had slightly higher levels on average) (3). This result approached statistical significance, which is pretty amazing, given the small sample size.

How does exercise reduce inflammation? One way may be by reducing centrally located fat. You may recall from our discussion in Part I that abdominal fat cells produce inflammatory factors. Furthermore, evidence is mounting that exercise also has direct effects on the expression of inflammatory genes, yet another method of reducing inflammation. In healthy volunteers, exercise turns off pro-inflammatory gene expression through DNA methylation, an on-off switch for genes which we will discuss in more detail later.

Exercise didn't only affect inflammation. Women who exercised also had better immune function. The investigators of the REHAB trial looked at the effects of exercise training on measurements of immune function. They measured natural killer cell (NK) cytotoxic activity in blood samples of the patients who participated in the exercise program compared to those who were in the control group. They found that the women who exercised had more effective NK activity, a key measure of immune function (4). Going back to our party analogy, the REHAB trial offers proof that exercise improves the "neighborhood" as well as the "police force".

But wait, there's more. Women who exercised also had lower levels of insulin-like growth factor and other related growth factors that have been proven to increase the growth of breast cancer cells (5). Going back again to our analogy, this is like cutting off the supply of beer and marijuana to the party.

So how does exercise work, biologically, to improve breast cancer outcomes? The data from this well performed randomized controlled trial indicates that it is multifactorial. Exercise works on all three major levels of tumor promotion. It improves the environment, the immune surveillance, and it reduces the tumor promoting growth factors. By looking at the biology behind the activity, we can see why and how exercise halts the unruly behavior of breast cancers.

As you can appreciate from this small study, it is often easier to prove a biological effect of an intervention than a "final readout effect" such as survival or reduction in recurrence. Having said that, even this small study proved an effect of exercise on a clinically important endpoint. The women in the exercise arm of the study had better fitness parameters such as heart rate. They also reported a better quality of life than those who were in the control arm (2).

♀ Key Study: Diet quality and inflammation

If elevated CRP is associated with worse survival and a high quality diet is associated with better survival, is a high quality diet linked to a lower CRP? This is the question that the HEAL investigators asked of their data.

In the HEAL study, 746 participants had measures of dietary intake scored for quality by the HEI-2005 index as well as serum CRP levels assayed (6). Breast cancer survivors with the highest quality diet (top quarter of the HEI-2005 scores, greater than 75) had significantly lower CRP levels than those with the lowest diet quality scores (less than 57). The average CRP concentration was 1.6 mg/L in those who consumed a quality diet vs 2.5 mg/L in those who consumed the worst quality diet.

Since a worse quality diet is associated with higher body mass, it could be that the elevated CRP was due to more body fat in those who ate a worse diet. As we discussed in Part I, higher BMI is associated with elevated CRP levels. The investigators factored this in by adjusting for BMI. The association between diet and CRP levels was maintained even after adjusting for BMI, meaning that it is not just fat that is accounting for the elevated CRP in those who consume a poor diet.

Exercise works hand in hand with diet, as we discussed in Part III. Exercise also reduces CRP. The HEAL investigators thus asked whether exercise affected the relationship between diet and CRP. They found that it does. Breast cancer survivors who reported engaging in any amount of exercise had lower CRP levels regardless of diet (CRP levels between 1.6 mg/L and 1.4 mg/L for the worst and best diets, respectively. These are not significantly different). However, women who did not exercise at all had significantly different CRP levels depending on diet quality; the average CRP level was 5.0 mg/L in those with the worst diet vs 2.5 mg/L in those who ate the best. We saw a similar relationship between diet and exercise earlier when looking at other outcomes. Exercise trumps diet. If you eat poorly, you can overcome the adverse effects by exercise. Of course, if you eat well and exercise, it's even better. These data suggest that reducing inflammation may be one of the ways this works.

♀ *Key Study: Dietary fats and inflammation*

In part III, we discussed the importance of the balance between omega-3 and omega-6 fatty acids. Let's look at how this might work from a biological standpoint. Studies related to heart disease in the general population have established that people who eat a diet higher in omega-3 polyunsaturated fatty acids have lower levels of inflammatory markers. Does the balance between omega-3 and omega-6 fatty acids affect inflammation levels in breast cancer survivors? If so, this could have major implications given the link between CRP and survival.

Investigators from the HEAL study looked at their data to see whether dietary fat intake was associated with inflammation, as measured by CRP levels. Diet reports from 633 women in the HEAL study were classified by omega-3 and omega-6 fatty acid intake. Diet was then correlated with CRP to measure inflammation.

There was a strong association between dietary fat intake and CRP levels (7). Breast cancer survivors who had higher intake of omega-6 compared to omega-3 fatty acids had higher CRP levels, indicating more inflammation. Roughly 40% of the women in the HEAL study had high-risk CRP levels. Women who were taking omega-3 supplements had the lowest omega-6:omega-3 ratios and also the lowest CRP levels. The risk of having a high CRP was 4.6 times higher in the breast cancer survivors who were in the top third of the omega-6:omega-3 ratio compared to those who were in the lowest omega-6:omega-3 ratio for diet and also took omega-3 supplements.

This study raises some provocative questions. How best to increase the omega-3 intake? Should we be taking fish oil supplements? Or is it more important to reduce the omega-6 intake, since that is the culprit linked to inflammation as well as reducing omega-3 metabolism? Should we be treating the inflammation with anti-inflammatory medications? Or are there other, potentially safer means of reducing inflammation, such as lifestyle behaviors? We don't have the answers yet.

💊 Key Study: Dietary fiber and inflammation

Another way to reduce inflammation via diet is to consume more fiber. In studies of the general population, higher intake of fiber is associated with lower levels of inflammatory markers. The HEAL investigators looked at their data to see whether increasing intake of fiber was associated with lower levels of inflammatory markers in breast cancer survivors.

In this group of 698 participants, the average CRP levels was 3.32 mg/L. It is relevant, and disappointing, to note that the average CRP in breast cancer survivors is already elevated (the definition of a high CRP in the general population is anything greater than 3 mg/L). However, the CRP levels were significantly lower in breast cancer survivors who consumed more fiber. Women who ate more than 15.5 grams of insoluble fiber per day had a nearly 50% reduction in the likelihood of having elevated CRP concentrations. Put another way, for every one-gram increase in fiber intake, the data predicts a 3-4% decrease in serum CRP levels (8).

How does fiber reduce CRP? No one knows for sure, but there are a few likely explanations. First, fiber helps to maintain a normal body weight, and, as we've seen, being overweight is associated with increased levels of inflammation. Another mechanism is the complex influence of fiber on several gut processes. Fiber has been associated with beneficial shifts in gut microbial composition, also known as gut flora. Gut microbes play an important role in immune function. The gut mucosa also produces many inflammatory mediators, so a beneficial and stabilizing effect of fiber may reduce this source of inflammation. Fiber is also full of micronutrients that can have a direct effect on the expression and function of inflammatory mediators. Fiber, particularly insoluble fiber, interferes with glucose absorption, which, in turn, affects insulin surges. The fact that the reduction in inflammatory markers was associated only with insoluble fiber in the HEAL study, and not soluble fiber, supports this idea.

Inflammation causes cancer-related fatigue

So far, the studies discussed above have investigated the link behind lifestyle behaviors and a biological endpoint – measures of inflammation. But this is still a step removed from an actual outcome. We already know that chronic inflammation is bad for our bodies. After all, you may have heard from the popular media that "silent inflammation is deadly". We also have seen that inflammation is associated with worse survival in breast cancer survivors. But survival is an end read-out of many factors. To dive more specifically into breast cancer related outcomes, several groups started looking at the link between inflammation and one important outcome: fatigue.

Fatigue is one of the most common, and most difficult complications of breast cancer treatment. Studies of long-term cancer survivors suggest that approximately a quarter to a third will experience persistent, debilitating fatigue for 10 years and longer after diagnosis and treatment (9). This has a negative impact on work, social relationships, mood, daily activities, and overall quality of life (10). Cancer-related fatigue is different than lack-of-sleep fatigue, with distinct mental, physical, and emotional components. As one group of investigators define it, cancer fatigue is "a state of overwhelming and sustained exhaustion and decreased capacity for physical and mental work that is not relieved by rest" (11). Studies conducted over the past decade have begun to elucidate the biological underpinnings of cancer-related fatigue: that inflammation is a primary cause of it (12).

To study the link between inflammation and fatigue in breast cancer survivors, experts in the study of fatigue turned their attention to *cancer-related fatigue*. Investigators from the University of California, Los Angeles Department of Psychology asked whether there was a link between inflammation and either fatigue, depression, or sleep disturbance in 103 breast cancer survivors who had recently completed treatment (13). By the end of treatment, more than 60% of participants reported significant problems with fatigue and sleep, and 25% had symptoms of depression.

Not surprisingly, fatigue was related to depressive symptoms, as well as sleep deprivation. However, when levels of inflammatory markers in the blood were correlated with symptoms, one of the markers, sTNF-R2, was associated with fatigue, but not with sleep deprivation or depression.

sTNF-R2 is the nomenclature for the "soluble tumor necrosis factor receptor 2". This molecule has long been associated with cancer, specifically, with treatment of cancer. When the tumor necrosis factor receptor is cleaved (processed), it releases this cleavage product as a soluble factor in the blood. Thus, we can measure the cleavage/processing of the tumor necrosis factor in blood by measuring levels of sTNF-R2. Furthermore, TNF-R2 undergoes cleavage when it is stimulated by the pro-inflammatory molecule TNF-alpha. Thus, blood levels of sTNF-R2 serve as a marker for TNF-alpha activity. TNF-alpha stands for "tumor necrosis factor-alpha". It is a highly inflammatory molecule that has been linked to tumor progression.

Why is all of this biology important? Because it demonstrates the link between a directly related to cancer-inflammation factor with fatigue. For the first time, this isn't looking like a global process, but more like a cancer-related process. The fact that this factor associated with *fatigue* and not with *sleep deprivation* or *depression* further indicates that this is related to cancer-associated fatigue.

The investigators wanted to delve further into the mechanisms of cancer-induced fatigue. To do so, they needed to separate out, as much as possible, the pathways of cancer-induced fatigue and cancer-related inflammation from the general milieu of cytokines in the body. They looked at the effect of treatment on sTNF-R2 and found that chemotherapy treatment was associated with higher levels of fatigue, and also with higher levels of sTNF-R2. The fact that they found no significant association between chemotherapy and blood levels of CRP (the general marker of inflammation related to worse outcomes in breast cancer survivors that we discussed in the last section) further indicates that the sTNF-R2:fatigue association is specific the cancer-induced fatigue as opposed to general inflammatory state-induced fatigue.

In fact, they had already shown a correlation between fatigue and levels of sTNF-R2 in breast cancer survivors (14). This was definitely looking like a "real" phenomenon, one that they could begin to investigate to determine how and why cancer-related inflammation is linked to fatigue, and, most importantly, what can be done about it.

Biology: Genetic risk for cancer-related fatigue

Knowing now that specific inflammatory molecules are associated with cancer-related fatigue in breast cancer survivors, these scientists next asked why some but not all breast cancer survivors develop fatigue. Postulating that a genetic susceptibility for fatigue may reside in the genes related to those specific inflammatory molecules, they looked to see whether differences in expression of the key players, TNF (tumor necrosis factor), ILB (interleukin beta), or IL-6 (interleukin 6) would correspond with fatigue (15).

While we all have the same number of chromosomes, we all carry different combinations of genes, so that each of us (except for identical twins) is genetically unique. Even identical twins have functional genetic differences, because genes are turned on or off during our lifetimes, but we'll get more to that in a bit. First, let's focus on the genetic differences that result from whether one carries a high-activity allele (version of the gene) or a low-activity allele.

That's what Julia Bower's group of scientists looked at. They investigated whether having a high activity vs low activity version of three of the main culprits in the cancer-related inflammatory pathway made a difference in the likelihood of experiencing cancer-related fatigue. And sure enough, it did. Breast cancer survivors who had high-expression alleles for the inflammatory mediators were more likely to experience fatigue. In fact, as the number of high-expressing alleles increased for the three inflammatory mediators measured, the greater the likelihood of fatigue, and the greater the severity of fatigue. In particular, high-expressing alleles of TNF and IL-6 were each independently associated with fatigue. The combination of high expression of all 3 (TNF, IL-6, and ILB) was associated not only with fatigue, but also with depression and memory complaints, aka chemobrain.

The converse was also true; breast cancer survivors who had low-expressing genetic alleles were at lower risk of developing fatigue. It appeared that there is, indeed, a genetic predisposition to the risk of severe cancer-related fatigue. Furthermore, it is linked to genes that encode proteins involved in inflammation. The biology was definitely becoming clear. Bower and her colleagues could even quantify the effect.

To establish a further link between inflammation and fatigue, Bower and colleagues looks at *transcriptional activity* of inflammatory mediators. Genes encode the instructions, but they are carried out by making a working copy blueprint (mRNA) that is then used to build the proteins (translation). When certain genes are "more active" they make more copies of their mRNA. This can be measured by a very powerful process called gene expression array. Bower's group used this technology to ask whether genes involved in inflammatory signals were actively making more "blueprints". They looked at NF-kB, and at the glucocorticoid responsive genes (16). The glucocorticoid receptor (GR) and NF-kB have a yin-yang relationship whereby the GR, as an anti-inflammatory signal inhibits pro-inflammatory NF-kB. The investigators tested their hypothesis that persistent cancer-related fatigue is associated with increased transcription of pro-inflammatory genes and decreased transcription of anti-inflammatory genes.

They divided their cohort of breast cancer survivors into those whose fatigue was considered severe based on validated fatigue questionnaire scoring systems or those who did not have severe fatigue. Then, they looked at levels of mRNA for NF-kB and GR related genes in the two groups. Sure enough, the women who had high levels of fatigue had a significantly higher level of pro- vs anti-inflammatory transcripts, about 5x higher, than those who were not fatigued.

The story of the genetic control of cancer fatigue gets even more interesting. Not only do we carry different genetic propensity to have higher or lower levels of pro-inflammatory molecules that are linked to fatigue, but we are also subject to modification of gene expression. Genes, whether high-activity alleles or low-activity alleles can also be turned on or off by a processed called "methylation". Basically, a chemical methyl group is attached to the start point for transcription (the first step of the process of translating the genetic code into an actual protein). This acts like a switch to turn the transcription of that gene off. We don't have all of our genes turned on all the time. They are carefully regulated so that they only turn on when they're supposed to (except, of course, cancer, which turns on genes for growth that aren't supposed to be on). So, typically, these pro-inflammatory genes are supposed to be turned off, or methylated, most of the time.

Now, armed with an understanding that fatigue is linked to production of pro-inflammatory molecules, and that breast cancer survivors who have more active pro-inflammatory genes or who have more copies of the "blueprints", or mRNA, for production of pro-inflammatory molecules have a greater susceptibility to fatigue, these investigators now turned to the question of how chemotherapy and radiotherapy cause fatigue.

Chemotherapy-treated breast cancer patients experience significantly more cancer-related fatigue than non-chemotherapy patients. Furthermore, chemotherapy is associated with increased markers of inflammation, including sTNF-R2 and IL-6 (17). Finally, chemotherapy and radiotherapy are known to affect DNA methylation, that "on/off" switch for gene expression. Therefore, another group of investigators built upon the foundation of Bower's work to see whether chemotherapy was associated with changes in methylation patterns of pro-inflammatory genes (18). They recruited 61 breast cancer patients, some who had had chemotherapy, and some who had not, and compared DNA methylation patterns between the two groups. Compared to those who did not receive chemotherapy, those treated with chemotherapy had reduced methylation in the promoters of genes involved in inflammatory responses. In other words, their pro-inflammatory genes were turned "on". This, in turn, correlated with higher levels of sTNF-R2 and IL-6. Furthermore, both decreased methylation and increased levels of pro-inflammatory proteins was associated with increased fatigue. Finally, some of these changes persisted at 6 months, indicating that specific genes may be involved in long-term fatigue in some patients in response to chemotherapy.

This body of work demonstrates that inflammation and fatigue are biologically linked. Cancer-related fatigue is likely manifested through elevated expression of specific pro-inflammatory markers, which occurs at a genetic level by either innate propensity for higher expression or through epigenetic manipulation of DNA methylation, via treatment or other environmental factors. This cutting edge research is just beginning to elucidate a fascinating example of gene-environment interaction. The good news is that we can often correct unfavorable gene-environment interactions. Thus, we have every hope that in the future we will understand how to correct debilitating effects of cancer via lifestyle practices. In Part V, we will see an example of this approach in action.

♀ *Key Study: Link between diet,*

inflammation, fatigue

Now that we have traced a link between inflammation and cancer related fatigue, let's look again at the data on diet to see whether inflammation that is linked to dietary habits is also linked to fatigue. Investigators from the HEAL study asked whether fatigue was greater amongst the women who had higher CRP than those with lower CRP levels (7).

Forty two of the women in the HEAL study were considered to have significant fatigue as measured by the Piper Fatigue Scale. This scale classifies fatigue into four categories: behavioral changes in activities due to fatigue, emotional meaning of fatigue, physical symptoms of fatigue, and emotional symptoms of fatigue. Vitality was also measured by another scoring system.

Both behavioral and sensory fatigue scores increased with higher CRP levels. When CRP scores were divided into three categories of low, middle, and high, the results showed that breast cancer survivors who had the highest levels of CRP were 2.4 times more likely to have significant fatigue than those in the lowest level. Those with an intermediate level of fatigue were 1.4 times more likely to have significant fatigue.

If inflammation, as measured by CRP levels, is associated with fatigue and omega-6:omega-3 ratio is associated with higher CRP, does the omega-6:omega-3 food intake correlate with fatigue? Yes, it does. The investigators found significant associations between amount of omega-6 fats eaten compared to omega-3 and fatigue. The association was particularly strong for the behavioral, sensory, and cognitive aspects of fatigue, as well as total fatigue.

This study links dietary intake of fat with levels of inflammation, and then levels of inflammation with increased fatigue. The study suggests that improving diet can improve fatigue as well as survival outcomes, but this remains to be proven by future studies. While we wait for the proof, the evidence from this study may further convince you to increase your omega-3 intake and decrease the omega-6 fatty acids in your diet.

Does inflammation cause cancer-related fatigue?

Although we have evidence that breast cancer survivors with higher levels of inflammatory markers have worse fatigue, this isn't necessarily proof that inflammation is a cause of worse outcomes in breast cancer. To prove that inflammation actually causes poorer outcomes, as opposed to being associated with poorer outcomes but not necessarily the causative factor, we would need to see a randomized, controlled clinical trial looking at outcomes in addition to biomarkers of inflammation.

But how do you randomize breast cancer survivors to high vs low inflammatory states to see whether there is a difference in outcomes based on levels of inflammation? Perhaps you can see how difficult it would be to design such a trial. It was done, and it worked. Read on for the answer to fatigue.

References: Part IV

1) Pierce BL, Ballard-Barbash R, Bernstein L et al. Elevated biomarkers of inflammation are associated with reduced survival among breast cancer patients. J Clin Oncology 2009; 27:3437-3444.

2) Courneya K, Mackey J et al. Randomized controlled trial of exercise training in postmenopausal breast cancer survivors: cardiopulmonary and quality of life outcomes. J Clin Oncol 2003; 21:1660-68.

3) Fairey A, Courneya K, Field C et al. Effect of exercise training on C-reacitve protein in postmenopausal breast cancer survivors: a randomized controlled trial. Brain, Behavior, and Immunity 2005; 10:381-88.

4)Fairey A, Courneya K et al. Randomized controlled trial of exercise training and blood immune function in postmenopausal breast cancer survivors. J Appl Physiol 2005; 98:1534-40.

5) Fairey A, Courneya K et al. Effects of exercise training on fasting insulin, insulin resistance, insulin-like growth factors, and IGF binding proteins in postmenopausal breast cancer survivors: a randomized controlled trial. Cancer Epidemiol Biomarkers, Prevention 2003; 12:721-7.

6) George S, Neuhoser M, Mayne S et al. Postdiagnosis diet quality is inversely related to a biomarker of inflammation among breast cancer survivors. Cancer Epideimol Biomarkers Prev 2010; 19:2220-8.

7) Alfano C, Imayama I, Neuhouser M et al. Fatigue, Imflammation, and omega-3 and omega-6 fatty acid intake among breast cancer survivors. J Clin Oncol 2012; 30:1280-1287.

8) Villasenor A, Ambs A, Ballard-Barbash R et al. Dietary fiber is associated with circulating concentrations of C-reactive protein in breast cancer survivors: the HEAL study. Br Cancer Res Treat 2011; 129:485-494.

9) Bower J, Ganz P, Desmond K et al. Fatigue in long-term breast carcinoma survivors: a longitudinal investigation. Cancer 2006; 106:751-8.

10) Bower J, Ganz P, Desmond K et al. Fatigue in breast cancer survivors: occurrence, correlates, and impact on quality of life. J Clin Oncol 2000; 18:743-53.

11) Cella D, Peterman A, Passik S et al. Progress toward guidelines for the management of fatigue. Oncology (Huting) 1998; 12:369-77.

12) Bower J and Lamkin D. Inflammation and cancer-related fatigue: Mechanisms, contributing factors, and treatment implications. Brain, Behavior, and Immunity 2013; 30:S48-S57.

13) Bower J, Ganz, P, Irwin M et al. Inflammation and behavioral symptoms after breast cancer treatment: do fatigue, depression, and sleep disturbance share a common underlying mechanism? J Clin Oncol 2011; 29:3517-22.

14) Bower J, Ganz P, Aziz N et al. Fatigue and proinflammatory cytokine activity in breast cancer survivors. Psychosom Med 2002; 64:604-11.

15) Bower J, Ganz P, Irwin M et al. Cytokine genetic variations and fatigue among patients with breast cancer. J Clin Oncol 2013; 31:1656-61.

16) Bower J, Ganz P, Irwin M et al. Fatigue and gene expression in human leukocytes: increased NF-kB and decreased glucocorticoid signaling in breast cancer survivors with persistent fatigue. Brain, Behavior, and Immunity 2011; 25:147-50.

17) Torres M, Pace, T, Liu T et al. Predictors of depression in breast cancer patients treated with radiation: role of prior chemotherapy and nuclear factor kappa B. Cancer 2013; 119:1951-59.

18) Smith A, Connelly K, Pace T et al. Epigenetic changes associated with inflammation in breast cancer patients treated with chemotherapy. Brain, Behavior, and Immunity 2014; 38:227-36.

Part V: Yoga

Did you know that women who practiced yoga after their diagnosis of breast cancer reduced their stress and fatigue?

Did you know that practicing yoga reduces inflammation and can improve your quality of life?

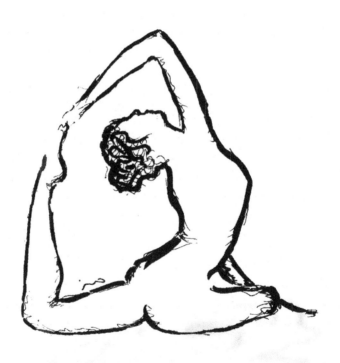

A treatment for fatigue and more

You may have noticed that nearly all of the data that we have discussed thus far has drawn associations between health behaviors and breast cancer outcomes. We have had very little randomized controlled trial data to draw on in order to show that those associations are actually causing the improved outcomes. In the rest of the book, we will be able to look at results from randomized controlled trials that do establish the causal connection between lifestyle behaviors and favorable outcomes. Let's begin to look at the data from randomized controlled trials of yoga by starting where we left off in the last part, on the inflammation: cancer related fatigue interaction.

We've seen that diet and exercise work hand in hand to reduce inflammation, and we left our discussion from the preceding section with the question of how one could design a randomized controlled trial to test whether a lifestyle factor would reduce inflammation and subsequently cause an improved outcome. When the group that established the biological underpinnings behind inflammation-induced cancer related fatigue in the preceding section wished to design a randomized controlled clinical trial to test the causality of this interaction, they could have chosen exercise or diet. After all, they knew what we now know, that an exercise program had been shown to reduce inflammation, and that diets that improve the omega-3: omega-6 fatty acid balance had been shown to reduce inflammation. However, there is yet another intervention that has a robust body of data behind it demonstrating that it reduces inflammation. And Bower's group chose this intervention to test their well-constructed biological hypothesis. What was this intervention? It was yoga.

Before delving into the data, let's clarify, what is yoga? Yoga is an ancient practice that includes breathing exercises (pranayana), postures (asanas), and meditation. It is meditative movement, focusing on developing bodily awareness. The root of the word yoga is "yoke", which some describe as yoga's intent of linking the mind and the body. Yoga is a mindful movement.

There are a few things that yoga is **not**. It is not pushing or straining. It is not a jock workout (although many athletes do use yoga for training). It is an inward-looking, "check in with your body" practice that should be done at your own pace and to your own abilities. We emphasize this because yoga poses can cause injury if not performed wisely. There are yoga programs that have been developed specifically for cancer survivors. These typically are gentle, avoid spine-stressing deep bends, and include a restorative component for deep relaxation. Oncology-based yoga programs are typically taught by instructors who are carefully aware of the limitations of bodies that have recently undergone surgery, may harbor metastatic disease, or are weaker as a result of treatment. As more and more cancer treatment centers recognize the benefits of yoga, these classes taught by oncology yoga instructors are becoming increasingly available.

Yoga, mindful movement, is a component of a larger program of mindfulness-based stress reduction. With both yoga and mindfulness-based stress reduction we have a wealth of well-performed randomized controlled clinical trials to discuss. We will start with the discussion of the clinical trials that separate out yoga as a single component. We will then turn to those that encompass yoga with within the context of full mindfulness programs in Part VI. This will allow us to be more specific about the benefits of yoga before we broaden our horizons to the benefits of mindfulness in general.

⚑ *Key Study: Yoga reduces inflammation*

The group that established the importance of inflammation in cancer-related fatigue implemented a randomized, controlled clinical trial to answer the question of whether yoga would treat inflammation-based fatigue in breast cancer survivors. Women who had persistent and severe cancer-related fatigue were randomized to a 12 week yoga class or a 12 week health education class (the "control" group). Blood samples were collected at the beginning, the end of the course, and 3 months after completion of the course to look at gene expression, inflammatory factors in the blood, and cortisol (a measure of stress). Naturally, they looked specifically at those factors that they had already identified as involved in the cancer fatigue-inflammation link.

First, they looked at whether yoga did, in fact, reduce inflammation. Their findings were impressive. This trial involved only 31 women, but the results showed a statistically significant effect of yoga on reducing inflammatory activity (1). To see clear biological changes in such a small group shows a **very** strong effect. Yoga significantly reduced the levels of the pro-inflammatory transcription factor NF-kB (discussed in our foray into science in Part IV), and, conversely, increased activity of the anti-inflammatory glucocorticoid receptor.

Furthermore, yoga had a significant effect in stabilizing levels of the pro-inflammatory sTNF-R2, whereas it increased in the control group. This proves that yoga reduces inflammation.

♥ Key Study: Yoga for fatigue

The study by Bower et al was designed to see whether fatigue, not just inflammation, could be reduced by yoga. Indeed, they found a statistically significant reduction in fatigue in the yoga group compared with the health education control group who didn't practice yoga (2). How much did the yoga help with the fatigue? Statisticians can crunch numbers to come up with an "effect size". In this study, they demonstrated a large effect, one that is considerably larger than the small to moderate effects seen with other interventions studied for cancer-related fatigue. You didn't have to be a statistician to ferret out the effect. By the three month follow-up, participants rated their fatigue low enough so that they no longer fell into the category of having significant post-treatment fatigue.

It is notable that the yoga group not only had steady improvement in fatigue from beginning to end of the program, but also that these effects persisted for three months afterward. Furthermore, yoga participants felt more confident about their ability to manage fatigue and its impact on their lives.

The investigators of this study asked another question as well. They asked whether those who did more yoga showed more effects than those who did less. Yes, more frequent practice produced larger benefits, both in fatigue and vitality as well as in the biological measurements of inflammation. For instance, a 10 minute per day increase in yoga practice was associated with a further 5-8% decrease in the levels of inflammatory markers.

This study was a rigorously designed study. It compared an intervention (yoga) against another intervention (an educational program such as those run by New Life *after* Cancer). The expectation was that only yoga would improve fatigue, but that both interventions may have psychological benefits, those associated with empowerment. This is exactly what the investigators found. Both interventions improved stress and depression.

For the 30% of breast cancer survivors who suffer debilitating fatigue, we now understand that it is related to unbridled inflammation. We also know that it can be corrected by expensive drugs? Maybe. But even better, by exercise. By yoga! By a lifestyle intervention that will also bring you improved sleep, improvement in hot flashes, improved immunity, and better quality of life (read on).

But what about those who don't suffer from fatigue? Does yoga reduce inflammatory signals in those who don't have a revved up inflammatory response? Another group of investigators asked that question by performing a randomized, controlled trial of 200 breast cancer survivors who were not selected on the basis of fatigue, but were selected from a group of all-comers. They had completed their treatment by at least several months, and then were randomly assigned to a 12 week yoga intervention (2x/week for 90 minutes, plus home practice) or a wait-list (control). Fatigue, vitality, depression, and inflammatory markers were measured at baseline, at the end of the 12 week course, and three months after the course was completed.

The group that was randomly assigned to the yoga practice had significantly less fatigue and more vitality than the control group (3). Furthermore, they had lower levels of the inflammatory factors IL-6, TNF-alpha, and IL-1. Importantly, these effects were even stronger with time; the improvements at three months after completion of the course were greater than those at the end of the course.

In aggregate, these randomized, controlled clinical trials demonstrate that yoga reduces inflammation and fatigue in breast cancer survivors, regardless of baseline fatigue or inflammatory states. Do you remember that decreased inflammation is associated with improved survival? Yoga is one of the most powerful practices breast cancer survivors can employ. It's proven by the highest level of evidence, the randomized controlled clinical trial.

♀ Key Study: Yoga improves quality of life

One of the very first randomized controlled trials of yoga in breast cancer survivors who had already completed therapy was performed at the University of Calgary. The investigators looked at physical and psychological benefits of yoga in 38 cancer survivors, 85% of whom were breast cancer survivors (4). Participants must have completed treatment at least three months prior to enrolling on the trial. The average time of completion of treatment before starting yoga program was five years. The program used was a 7-week modified Iyengar yoga, with the asanas modified to be particularly gentle. A battery of self-report questionnaire instruments was used to compare pretreatment to immediately after completion of the seven week course.

Physical fitness improved modestly in both the control group and the yoga group. It is notable that many of the patients in the control group also engaged in exercise programs. There were, however significant improvements in the yoga group over the control group in emotional functioning as well as global improvement in quality of life. There were also improvements in levels of tension and, interestingly, decreased shortness of breath.

For breast cancer survivors who struggle with low mood, yoga may be particularly beneficial (5). A study of restorative yoga (a style of very gentle, relaxing yoga) vs wait list control in 44 breast cancer survivors, including those under treatment, showed particular benefit of this gentle, compassionate form of yoga for those who started at a lower state of emotional well-being.

The largest and most prominent study was published in the highly prestigious Journal of Clinical Oncology in 2007 (6). This well-performed study randomized 128 breast cancer survivors (nearly half still undergoing treatment) to yoga vs wait list control, and asked whether yoga improved quality of life, fatigue, mood, or spiritual well-being. The program consisted of once weekly yoga for 12 weeks. Unlike the last two studies, which were very specific in their inclusion criteria, this study included patients from a medically diverse group. Furthermore, they were an ethnically diverse group, with a majority of African American or Hispanic ethnicity. The results of yoga differed depending on whether participants were still undergoing treatment or not. For those who were finished with treatment, a significant improvement in quality of life was seen compared to the control group. Similar changes were seen with emotional, social, and spiritual well-being. Yoga practitioners also were less likely to experience distress, anxiety or sadness, or irritability than those who were not in the yoga group.

♀ *Key Study: Yoga improves sleep*

Another large, randomized controlled trial was also published in the Journal of Clinical Oncology. Involving 410 cancer survivors (75% breast cancer) who had completed all treatment, it was a multi-center study led by the University of Rochester, spanning institutions from California to New York (7). The study randomized breast cancer survivors to a 4-week yoga program using gentle Hatha and Restorative yoga, meditation, and breathing (the Yoga for Cancer Survivors program) vs standard care follow-up (including prescribing sleep medication).

The specific question posed in this study was whether yoga would improve sleep. As we discussed in Part IV, sleep disturbance (which is different from fatigue) is very common amongst cancer survivors, and significantly affects function, quality of life, mood, and depression.

The study showed that yoga improved sleep disturbance, specifically improving the quality of sleep, decreasing daytime dysfunction as a result of sleep loss, and waking up in the middle of the night. Yoga participants experienced large improvements in sleep quality (effect size 0.62) while the control group did not. This is particularly impressive since the yoga participants also reduced their use of sleep medication by 21% per week. Importantly, sleep was improved even in those who did not start with much in the way of sleep disturbance. However, those who had more than one hour of wakefulness in the middle of the night, very poor sleep efficiency, or both, were the ones who improved the most.

This study should pave the way for additional studies that would specifically compare yoga to other forms of sleep therapy (for example, cognitive behavioral therapy, guided imagery, etcetera). However, while we wait for those to determine which intervention is most effective, it is nice to know that practicing yoga is something that you can do to combat the sleep demons.

♀ Key Study: Yoga for weight loss

Another study looked at the effects of a 6-month long yoga practice in overweight breast cancer survivors (8). This study involved 63 women in a lengthy studio- and home-based program that proved to be unfeasible because it was too difficult to recruit participants to such a long intervention. However, despite the difficulties with enrollment, the participants who did enroll tended to complete the program.

The difficulty with recruitment caused the study to take too long to meet the accrual goals. It closed early. Despite this, the study demonstrated that quality of life and fatigue were improved in the yoga group as compared to the wait-list control group.

The primary endpoint of the study was weight loss, which didn't improve with yoga. However, the women who practiced yoga trimmed on average three cm off their waist-lines. Thus, it looks as though yoga isn't a good way to go about casting off those extra pounds. But if the important part of weight control is really a reduction in the metabolically active abdominal fat, this small study suggests that yoga may benefit overweight breast cancer survivors.

♀ Key Study: Yoga improves hot flashes

An early randomized controlled trial of yoga in post-treatment breast cancer survivors looked at the effects of an eight week course of yoga vs wait-list control on hot flashes in 37 women (9). The yoga program was developed at Duke University, and dubbed the "Yoga of Awareness Program". In addition to yoga, it included meditation and discussion time; however, the emphasis was on asanas (poses), so was not considered a full mindfulness program.

The group that received the yoga program had greater improvements in hot flashes compared to the waiting women. The women who practiced yoga had on average a quarter fewer hot flashes per day by the completion of the course, whereas the women who were waiting had no decrease. Furthermore, the yoga practitioners were less bothered by the hot flashes that they did still experience, perhaps because they were milder (the severity was reduced by about a quarter in the yoga group as well), or perhaps they were better tolerated, or both. They also had improvements in joint pain, fatigue, sleep disturbance, and vigor. Importantly, when compared three months after the yoga program was over, these benefits persisted.

This was a small study, and published in a minor journal, so it didn't necessarily get a lot of attention, but it was a well-conducted study and paved the way for future investigation. This is also an important study because it is one of the few studies of any type of intervention that shows an improvement in hot flashes. What a relief!

♀ *Key Study: Yoga during treatment*

Although our focus in this book is specifically on the effects of lifestyle interventions after treatment, there are a handful of studies that look at effects of yoga during treatment that we think are worth mentioning.

Yoga has been shown to reduce chemotherapy-associated nausea and vomiting in a randomized, controlled clinical trial. Sixty-two breast cancer survivors undergoing chemotherapy were randomly allocated to a yoga practice intervention or supporting therapy, specifically to see whether yoga would improve nausea and vomiting (10). Yoga significantly reduced post-chemotherapy nausea frequency and intensity. It also reduced anticipatory nausea and vomiting (when you get sick even before treatment because of the memory of the last treatment).

In the randomized trial mentioned in the previous section, we pointed out that the benefits of yoga were not seen in patients who are undergoing treatment. But one problem was that patients who are undergoing radiotherapy did not adhere to their yoga program. This was very different in a study from India, where patients received their yoga classes in the radiotherapy clinic. In this trial of yoga vs supportive therapy in 88 women with early stage breast cancer who were undergoing radiation therapy, patients were much more likely to complete their yoga sessions (11). Yoga sessions consisted of a one-hour class three times weekly while they were in the clinic for radiotherapy. Women assigned to the control group received one-hour counseling sessions. The primary question was whether there would be any difference in quality of life or mood, measured by well-validated questionnaires that specifically measure these factors. Women in the yoga group had a significant improvement in positive mood, decrease in negative mood, improvement in emotional function, and in cognitive function. They also had better physical activity, improved social relations, and better overall quality of life. Furthermore, the magnitude of the effect of yoga was not small. The benefits of yoga were quite clear.

Another recent randomized controlled trial of yoga during radiotherapy asked whether yoga would improve overall quality of life, as well as fatigue, in breast cancer patients undergoing treatment. The investigators of this study went a step further and compared yoga not only to a control group receiving supportive care, but also to a control group who underwent stretching exercises, but not the meditative aspects of yoga (12).

The study showed that yoga improved strength, reduced fatigue, and improved quality of life, when compared to either the supportive care control group or the stretching-intervention group. Furthermore, the benefits persisted with time, measured at three months after completion of radiotherapy.

Biology: Effects of yoga

The investigators who studied yoga during radiotherapy asked some interesting biological questions, with provocative results. Would yoga influence biologic measurements of stress? One way to measure stress is to look at levels of cortisol, a stress hormone, in the saliva. It's a bit complicated, since levels vary drastically between people and also vary depending on the time of day, but researchers have learned that the changes in cortisol levels over time correlate with health outcomes, including breast cancer outcomes. The investigators of the trial of yoga vs stretching wanted to see whether the mindfulness aspects of yoga would improve stress as measured by cortisol levels.

Yes, they did. The higher levels of cortisol, generally associated with the stress of diagnosis and treatment, decreased much more rapidly in the women who practiced yoga compared to those who received counseling sessions or stretching exercise sessions (12). This study confirms that yoga can reduce physical stress levels as well as stress measured by questionnaires.

But there's also another fascinating effect of yoga on biological responses to radiotherapy. We know that radiation induces genotoxic stress, that is, it causes a small amount of DNA damage outside of the radiation treatment field. A randomized, controlled trial of yoga vs supportive care during radiotherapy allowed investigators to ask whether yoga had any effect on this toxic stress DNA damage (13).

DNA damage was seen after radiotherapy in the lymphocytes (white blood cells) of both the control patients and the yoga practitioners, but it was significantly lower in those who practiced yoga (14.5% lower). Furthermore, in addition to a decrease in genotoxic stress, yoga also reduced symptoms of stress; women in the yoga group had better scores on the "perceived stress" survey. Patients who were randomized to the yoga practice group had a 25% decrease in their symptoms of stress, whereas the control group that received counseling experienced no decrease in DNA-damage stress from before to after completion of radiotherapy.

Finally, a study from Washington State University looked at the effects of Iyengar yoga on fatigue and stress in 18 breast cancer survivors (14). This small study is intriguing because of the efforts to measure stress levels biologically using measurement of the stress hormone, cortisol. This study was too small and the numbers too variable to say with much confidence that the results are firm, but it did show an intriguing reduction in cortisol in the group that participated in yoga. Furthermore, despite small numbers of participants, the investigators found a decrease in fatigue that supports the contention that yoga may improve well-being via reductions in stress response that contribute to fatigue, as well as the inflammation-based pathways we discussed in Part IV.

♥ *Key Study: Meta-analysis of yoga studies*

You can see from the studies that yoga has a wide range of benefits the breast-cancer survivors. Just how much of a benefit? How large is the effect? This question can be answered with a meta-analysis. A meta-analysis is a larger analysis of many randomized clinical trials. The data from each of the trials is combined, so that one may get an overall view of the end result of many different studies. This allows the statisticians to calculate an *effect size*. In other words, what's the number on the difference between yoga and all of the other control interventions? How effective is it? This also allows us to compare the benefit of one thing to the benefit of something completely different. For example, kidney dialysis is considered to have a large effect compared to no dialysis. We can then qualify various interventions into categories of having a large, moderate, or minimal effect.

There have been at least 15 well-conducted, randomized-controlled clinical trials investigating the benefits of yoga for breast cancer patients, where yoga was the main focus of the intervention and not a part of more comprehensive mindfulness-based stress relief programs. Some trials were large, and some were small. The yoga programs varied from weekly to daily sessions from 30 to 120 minutes per session, and lasted from 4 weeks to 6 months. Some of the trials targeted patients who were undergoing treatment, while others included only women who had completed their full course of treatment, or a combination of both. Some of the studies compared yoga to other interventions, such as educational survivorship sessions, counseling, expressive therapy sessions, or other exercise classes.

A meta-analysis of these studies was performed to provide the overall view of the benefits, as well at the magnitude of those benefits (15). The meta-analysis showed that yoga **significantly** reduces distress, anxiety, and depression in breast cancer survivors (greater than 70% reduction). It also **moderately** improves fatigue, health-related quality of life, and emotional and social function (50-70% improvement).

In the preceding discussion of diet and exercise, we had to rely on nonrandomized trials to provide the data. In the case of yoga and mindfulness-based stress reduction, we have a wealth of randomized controlled clinical trials from which to draw our conclusions. This level of evidence is much stronger. Randomized controlled clinical trials provide Level 1 evidence for the effectiveness of the tested intervention. This is what constitutes proof. Practice patterns are changed based on Level 1 evidence of efficacy. Yoga has been proven in randomized controlled trials to have a wide range of benefits in breast cancer survivors, ranging from improvements in post treatment side effects to global improvements in general quality of life. The data speaks for itself. Insurance companies should put their money on lifestyle interventions of yoga and mindfulness-based intervention stress reduction. So should all of us.

Prescription: Part V

Practice yoga three times weekly

The evidence:

- Randomized controlled trials show that yoga improves fatigue and inflammation in both severely fatigued and non-fatigued breast cancer survivors (2, 3).
- Randomized controlled trials show that yoga improves mood, emotional functioning, and quality of life (5, 6).
- A randomized controlled trial shows that yoga improves sleep in breast cancer survivors compared to usual care, with a large and clinically relevant effect (3).
- A randomized, controlled trial shows that yoga improves hot flashes (9).
- A randomized controlled trial of yoga in breast cancer patients undergoing radiotherapy shows that yoga reduces stress symptoms and cortisol levels. Yoga also reduced genotoxic damage (4, 5).
- A meta-analysis of 13 randomized, controlled clinical trials show that yoga significantly reduces distress, anxiety, and depression in breast cancer survivors (>70% reduction compared to control arm). It also **moderately** improves fatigue, health-related quality of life, and emotional and social function (50-70% improvement compared to control) (15).

Lolly's yoga story

On the same day in 2010 that I began a weight loss program, I attended my first yoga class ever, encouraged by the New Life *after* Cancer retreat. Yoga was offered through the Comprehensive Cancer Support Program at the University of North Carolina. Almost immediately I knew that I had found a form of exercise that I would love and would pursue. I was not very good at first when everything was new, despite the fact that I am fairly limber, but I was determined to stick with it.

There were three classes offered each week, and I went to all of them. My teaching schedule permitted morning yoga classes, then I would go to the law school after class. There were two teachers both trained in gentle yoga for cancer survivors. I liked both of them, but one of them was spectacular. Doreen Stein-Seroussi is an amazing teacher with whom I continue to study. Doreen has the ability to work with and encourage someone brand new to yoga while at the same time challenge experienced yoga students. As I began to learn the names of the poses and perfect them to the best of my ability, I realized what yoga was doing for my body. I became stronger and my balance improved. Doreen refers to the flows that we practice as moving meditation, and I believe it. I am not the best at meditating since my mind goes several miles an hour, but concentrating on the poses through a flow totally occupies my mind and makes me live in the now. Further, the breathing helps to calm my mind, and I use the breathing techniques in my daily life.

Another cancer support program offered yoga classes with Doreen and I began to attend that class also, practicing four times weekly. One class was cancelled, so I am back down to three classes per week. I would go every day, if it were offered! Now that I am retired, yoga classes structure my days.

I would like to get much better at yoga now that I have practiced for six years, but realistically, it is likely to be only incremental. While I have only one real physical limitation, a bad knee from surgery following a skiing accident in 1978, I am also 71 years old. So, as I learn more and strive to get better, my aging body pushes against much improvement. But I am determined to keep trying! I am brave and will try almost anything in yoga. Not that I can do everything, but I will try!

Yoga has improved my life tremendously. I thrive on both the mental and the physical aspects of yoga. I try to push myself a little further each class, and I definitely have improved. I was totally unable to do planks when I first tried, and now they are easy. I have worked hard to do crows, and now can do them. My muscles are much stronger, and, after a lifetime with a flat butt, I now have a rear end, and I am pretty proud of it!

I wish I had come to yoga when I was younger, but I do plan to continue to practice it for the rest of my life.

Self-Assessment: Part V

How is your energy & mood?

Yoga offers many benefits to breast cancer survivors. However, some of the greatest benefits are in reducing fatigue, whether immune related or due to sleep deprivation. Fully 30% of breast cancer survivors qualify as significantly fatigued. How do you rate on fatigue? You can gauge yourself, if you like, using this PIPER fatigue assessment form, a revised version of the questionnaires that Bower's group used.

Piper Fatigue Scale-12 (PFS-12)

Directions Please circle the number which best describes the fatigue you are experiencing **IN THE PAST 4 WEEKS**

1 To what degree is the fatigue you are feeling interfering with your ability to complete your work or school activities?

0	1	2	3	4	5	6	7	8	9	10
None										A great deal

2 Overall, how much is the fatigue which you are experiencing interfering with your ability to engage in the kind of activities you enjoy?

0	1	2	3	4	5	6	7	8	9	10
None										A great deal

> **ALTERNATIVE WORDING for #2.**
> ***NOTE: THIS ITEM HAS NOT BEEN TESTED.**
>
> *To what degree is the fatigue you are feeling interfering with your ability to do the activities you enjoy?*
>
> | 0 | 1 | 2 | 3 | 4 | 5 | 6 | 7 | 8 | 9 | 10 |
> |---|---|---|---|---|---|---|---|---|---|---|
> | *None* | | | | | | | | | | *A great deal* |

3 How would you describe the degree of intensity or severity of the fatigue which you are experiencing?

0	1	2	3	4	5	6	7	8	9	10
Mild										Severe

4 To what degree would you describe the fatigue which you are experiencing as being:

0	1	2	3	4	5	6	7	8	9	10
Pleasant										Unpleasant

5. To what degree is the fatigue you are feeling now interfering with your ability to engage in sexual activity?

None   A Great Deal

1   2   3   4   5   6   7   8   9   10

6. Overall, how much is the fatigue which you are now experiencing interfering with your ability to engage in the kind of activities you enjoy doing?

None   A Great Deal

1   2   3   4   5   6   7   8   9   10

7. How would you describe the degree of intensity or severity of the fatigue which you are experiencing now?

Mild   Severe

1   2   3   4   5   6   7   8   9   10

8. To what degree would you describe the fatigue which you are experiencing now as being?

Pleasant   Unpleasant

1   2   3   4   5   6   7   8   9   10

9. To what degree would you describe the fatigue which you are experiencing now as being?

Agreeable   Disagreeable

1   2   3   4   5   6   7   8   9   10

10. To what degree would you describe the fatigue which you are experiencing now as being?

Protective   Destructive

1   2   3   4   5   6   7   8   9   10

11. To what degree would you describe the fatigue which you are experiencing now as being?

Positive   Negative

1   2   3   4   5   6   7   8   9   10

12. To what degree would you describe the fatigue which you are experiencing now as being:

Normal   Abnormal

1   2   3   4   5   6   7   8   9   10

13. To what degree are you now feeling:

Strong   Weak

1   2   3   4   5   6   7   8   9   10

14. To what degree are you now feeling:

Awake   Sleepy

1   2   3   4   5   6   7   8   9   10

15. To what degree are you now feeling:

Lively   Listless

1   2   3   4   5   6   7   8   9   10

16. To what degree are you now feeling:

Refreshed   Tired

1   2   3   4   5   6   7   8   9   10

17. To what degree are you now feeling:

Energetic   Unenergetic

1   2   3   4   5   6   7   8   9   10

18. To what degree are you now feeling:

Patient   Impatient

1   2   3   4   5   6   7   8   9   10

19. To what degree are you now feeling:

Relaxed   A Great Deal

1   2   3   4   5   6   7   8   9   10

Self-Assessment

20. To what degree are you now feeling:

Exhilarated   Depressed

1   2   3   4   5   6   7   8   9   10

21. To what degree are you now feeling:

Able to Concentrate   Unable to Concentrate

1   2   3   4   5   6   7   8   9   10

22. To what degree are you now feeling:

Able to Remember   Unable to Remember

1   2   3   4   5   6   7   8   9   10

23. To what degree are you now feeling:

Able to Think Clearly   Unable to Think Clearly

1   2   3   4   5   6   7   8   9   10

24. Overall, what do you believe is _most_ directly contributing to or causing your fatigue?

_____

_____

25. Overall, the _best_ thing you have found to relieve your fatigue is: _____

_____

_____

26. Is there anything else you would like to add that would describe your fatigue better to us?

_____

_____

27. Are you experiencing any other symptoms right now? _____

_____

_____

Another area where yoga really shines is in improving mood. The scale that was used to measure mood in many of the yoga studies is the POMS (profile of mood states). This tool is fairly complicated, you can learn more at: http://www.immpact.org/static/meetings/Immpact4/backg round/Haythornthwaite.pdf. An easier one to use is the Positive and Negative Affect Scale (PANAS). If you wish, you can see where you fit on the scale, and to follow your progress after you have practice yoga for a period of two to three months.

Worksheet 3.1   The Positive and Negative Affect Schedule (PANAS; Watson et al., 1988)

PANAS Questionnaire

This scale consists of a number of words that describe different feelings and emotions. Read each item and then list the number from the scale below next to each word. **Indicate to what extent you feel this way right now, that is, at the present moment *OR* indicate the extent you have felt this way over the past week (circle the instructions you followed when taking this measure)**

1 Very Slightly or Not at All	2 A Little	3 Moderately	4 Quite a Bit	5 Extremely

_____ 1. Interested		_____ 11. Irritable
_____ 2. Distressed		_____ 12. Alert
_____ 3. Excited		_____ 13. Ashamed
_____ 4. Upset		_____ 14. Inspired
_____ 5. Strong		_____ 15. Nervous
_____ 6. Guilty		_____ 16. Determined
_____ 7. Scared		_____ 17. Attentive
_____ 8. Hostile		_____ 18. Jittery
_____ 9. Enthusiastic		_____ 19. Active
_____ 10. Proud		_____ 20. Afraid

Scoring Instructions:

Positive Affect Score: Add the scores on items 1, 3, 5, 9, 10, 12, 14, 16, 17, and 19. Scores can range from 10 – 50, with higher scores representing higher levels of positive affect. Mean Scores: Momentary = 29.7 $(SD = 7.9)$; Weekly = 33.3 $(SD = 7.2)$

Negative Affect Score: Add the scores on items 2, 4, 6, 7, 8, 11, 13, 15, 18, and 20. Scores can range from 10 – 50, with lower scores representing lower levels of negative affect. Mean Score: Momentary = 14.8 $(SD = 5.4)$; Weekly = 17.4 $(SD = 6.2)$

Call to Action: Part V

In addition to your healthy eating habits and regular exercise, we encourage you to add yoga. A regular practice of yoga three times a week can count as part of your exercise regimen.

How do you find the right yoga program? Look first to see if there is a cancer center program in your area. Look to see whether there are yoga courses for retirees. You will probably be more likely to find the type of yoga course that the studies we've discussed used in a community center than in a gym. Finally, there are many good resources that are available for practice at home. Again, look for those DVDs and online programs that come from cancer centers and use the yoga programs that have been proven to provide the benefit.

Finding the right yoga program might take some searching. You have to start somewhere, but then use your judgment to determine whether the yoga class you have just tried is right for you. It should be peaceful. It should be gentle. Remember, yoga is exercise, but it is not meant to be a work-out that hurts you. Use your judgment.

If you find that yoga isn't a good fit for you, you might try other forms of mindful movement. Tai Chi is one such possibility. Indeed, a recently published randomized controlled trial shows that Tai Chi also reduces inflammation in breast cancer survivors.

As with our other calls to action, and the healthy habits you have developed from heeding those, we urge you to track your yoga practice. Add that to your healthy habits journal, and when you have practiced for two to three months, retake the mood and fatigue questionnaires. We bet that you will be delighted with what you see. Of course, by that time you will already feel it.

References: Part V

1) Bower J, Greendale G, Crosswell A et al. Psychoneuroendocrinology 2014; 43:20-29.

2) Bower J, Garet D, Sternlieb B et al. Yoga for persistent fatigue in breast cancer survivors: a randomized controlled trial. Cancer 2012; 118:3766-75.

3) Kiecolt-Glaser J, Bennett J, Andridge R et al. Yoga's impact on inflammation, mood, and fatigue in breast cancer survivors: a randomized controlled trial. J Clin Oncology 2014; 32:1040-49

4) Culos-Reed, Psycho-oncology 15:891-7, 2006).

5) Danhauer S, Mihalko S, Russell G et al. Restorative yoga for women with breast cancer: findings from a randomized pilot study. Psycho-oncology 2009; 18:360 68.

6) Moadel A, Shah C, Rosett J et al. Randomized controlled trial of yoga among a multiethnic sample of breast cancer patients: effects on quality of life. J Clin Oncol 2007; 25:4387-95.

7) Mustian K, Sprod L, Janelsins M et al. Mutlicenter, randomized controlled trial of you for sleep quality among cancer survivors. J Clin Oncology 2013; 26:3233-41.

8) Littman AL Support Care Cancer, 2012, 20:267-77).

9) Carson J, Carson K, Porter L et al. Yoga of awareness program for menopausal symptoms in breast cancer survivors: results from a randomized trial. Support Care Cancer 2009; 17:1301-9.

10) Raghavendra R, Nagarathna R, Nagendra H et al. Effects of an integrated yoga program me on chemotherapy-induced nausea and emesis in breast cancer patients. European J of Cancer Care 2007; 16:462-74.

11) Vadiraja H, Ral M, Nagarathna R et al. Effects of yoga program on quality of life and affect in early breast cancer patients undergoing adjuvant radiotherapy; a randomized controlled trial. Complementary Therapies in Medicine 2009; 17:274-80.

12) Chandwani K, Perkins G, Nagendra H et al. Randomized, controlled trial of yoga in women with breast cancer undergoing radiotherapy. J Clin Oncology 2014; 32;1058-65.

13) Banerjee B, Vadiraj H, Ram A et al. Effects of an integrated yoga program in modulating psychological stress and radiation-

induced genotoxic stress in breast cancer patients undergoing radiotherapy. Integrative Cancer Therapies 2007; 6:242-50.

14) Banasik J, American Adademy of Nurse Practitioners 2011, 23:135-142).

15) Buffart L, van Uffelen J, Riphagen I et al. Physical and psychosocial benefits of yoga in cancer patients and survivors, a systematic review and meta-analysis of randomized controlled trials. BMC Cancer 2012; 12:559-72.

Part VI: Mindfulness Based Stress Reduction

Did you know that women who practiced mindfulness based stress reduction after their diagnosis of breast cancer improved their symptoms of emotional distress?

Did you know that mindfulness based stress reduction improves your overall quality of life and reduces stress?

Did you know that mindfulness based stress reduction improves hot flashes and loss of libido?

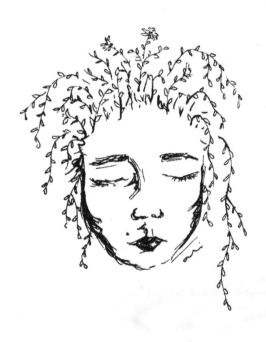

What is mindfulness-based stress reduction?

In Part V, we pointed out that yoga is an important component of a larger program, that of mindfulness-based stress reduction (MBSR). We had separated out the studies that looked specifically at yoga, but we will now turn to those studies that investigate the benefits of mindfulness-based stress reduction, which includes yoga, for breast cancer survivors. As with yoga, we are fortunate to have a robust body of randomized controlled clinical trials from which we can draw firm conclusions as to the benefit of mindfulness-based stress reduction as the actual cause of those benefits.

What does "mindfulness" mean? The Mental Health Foundation defines mindfulness succinctly: "It is a way of paying attention. It means consciously bringing awareness to our experience, in the present moment, without making judgements about it." Scientists of mindfulness explain further. "Most of the time, people are on 'automatic pilot', caught up in their experience and reacting automatically, especially when feeling stressed. Staying consciously aware of what is happening, that is, being mindful, allows people to observe and accept what they are currently experiencing, in their bodies, minds and the world around them. This provides opportunities for individuals to make more considered decisions about how to respond to what is happening" (1).

Mindfulness empowers. The investigators of one of the studies that we will discuss describe, "The value of mindfulness-based interventions for survivors of cancer is potentially multifaceted. The emphasis is not on changing the situation; rather, skill taught through mindfulness practice help participants change their way of relating to given life situations. MBSR helps facilitate development of positive emotional regulation strategies such as acceptance and gently extinguishes unhelpful strategies. As participants allow graduated exposure to feared thoughts and feelings during meditation practice, cultivated in an accepting and nonjudgmental environment, feared stimuli lose much of their power. The result is often a sense of heightened control, calm, peace, and serenity, even in the face of the many uncontrollable elements of cancer" (8).

Mindfulness-based stress reduction is a health and wellness program that was designed by John Kabat-Zinn at Massachusetts General Hospital in Boston to cultivate mindfulness as a healing approach for patients with chronic illness. Drawing on ancient practices of meditation, body awareness, and movement, he adapted these active Eastern practices to create a program for Western medicine and healthcare (1). The results were not short of amazing. He was able to prove significant benefits of his eight week program for patients with chronic pain, emotional injuries, and cancer. MBSR programs have now spread to many institutions throughout the United States and Europe, and are acknowledged as a proven therapeutic tool for a wide range of illnesses.

As the name implies, MBSR programs help people to deal with stress, whether the stress of chronic pain, or the stress of dealing with cancer. The effect of stress on cancer outcomes has been a hot topic for quite some time. It has been hampered somewhat by a lack of well validated studies, but that is changing markedly. As we touched on in the last chapter, stress can be biologically measured to some extent by looking at levels of cortisol in the blood. Stress can also be reproducibly measured by survey questionnaires. This has led to the ability to objectively study the effect of stress reduction interventions.

There are many different aspects to the practice of MBSR, but they all have in common the underlying theme of focusing attention and awareness on the mental (the thoughts) and the physical (the body). Yoga, meditation, and imagery are the three main tools in the MBSR toolkit. They are similar, but not interchangeable. They are best used in concert, as each adds a slightly different dimension to the others.

The distinction between yoga and MBSR is subtle. Both are technically meditative forms. Yoga is a meditative movement that focuses more on the external, the movement of the body. MBSR programs focus on the internal, the calling of the mind. Yoga is one component of a MBSR program. You can think of the MBSR programs as being a broader picture, one that focuses both on internal quieting of the mind as well as external connection with the body.

MBSR programs typically include yoga poses along with the meditation and visualization practices. We don't yet know which of these components of MBSR programs are responsible for the beneficial effects, but there are a number of studies that look specifically at the effects of yoga. We discussed those in the last chapter, where we distinguished those studies that looked at the effects of the asanas, the yoga poses, not at the effects of programs that include also a major meditative component. We saw that yoga has strong effects on fatigue, sleep, mood, and overall improvement in quality of life.

As we review the data for MBSR, we would offer this oversimplification: MBSR helps predominantly with emotional-psychological aspects of cancer recovery, yoga with dealing with the physical effects of diagnosis and treatment. They work hand in hand in a wonderfully complementary way, as do diet and exercise.

The most widely used MBSR program in the United States, at least in the healthcare setting, is still the program developed by Jon Kabat-Zinn. His excellent book, *Full Catastrophe Living: How to Cope with Stress, Pain and Illness Using Mindfulness Meditation,* continues to be a bestseller more than a decade after it was written (2). We owe credit to him for the recent revolution in the acceptance of mind-body practices as a validated and *bona fide* form of treatment for many physical ailments. There are many well-performed clinical trials that prove the benefit of MBSR-based rest reduction for a wide range of health ailments, including breast cancer.

How helpful is MBSR for breast cancer survivors? Let's take a look at the data.

The MBSR program

A review of the program used by the Moffitt Cancer Center study which we will discuss in the next section gives an excellent taste of what a MBSR course conveys.

During the first week, an introduction to meditation is taught, using a body scan procedure. The body scan is a systematic method of checking in with every part of your body to assay for how it feels, and teaching deep relaxation and concentration in the process.

In week two, visualization and awareness of breathing are taught, deepening conscious attention to typically ignored body processes.

In week three, participants are guided to gain an understanding of one's reaction to a pleasant event or a stressful event, focusing on how the body tenses or relaxes. Yoga is introduced at this time.

During the fourth week, the relationship between response and reaction are connected to a better understanding of the underlying thought process.

During week five, participants expand their field of awareness to allow for modification of stress inducing patterns, and continue to develop their awareness so that they can opt to change any stress-inducing reactions. Through meditation, awareness is extended from body sensations to thoughts and feelings.

In the final week, participants develop their own practice plan for the future. In this way, the course provides education related to relaxation, meditation and the mind-body connections, guides a practice of meditation, and incorporates discussion between participants that heightens awareness of benefits and barriers to developing a mindfulness practice.

Longer programs (like the Kabat-Zinn protocol) span eight weeks and incorporate a full day or weekend retreat, which intensifies the meditative components, including silent meditation.

Mind-body-emotional axis

The goal of mindfulness based stress reduction is achievement of a state of mental and physical wellbeing. By developing awareness of how we feel, both mentally and physically, we can learn to accept that which we cannot change and to change thoughts and habits that do not serve us well. The end result is the ability to create a positive emotional state. This is what the data shows.

Happiness, joy, love, gratefulness are positive emotional states. Anger, fear, anxiety, hatred are negative emotional states. These are measured in the studies that we will discuss in the next sections by using a series of validated survey instruments, that is, questionnaires. You can try it yourself in the "Self-Assessment" section at the end of this chapter.

Emotions are the conduit between the mind and the body. Research is just now scratching the surface of how our brains function, let alone the interactions between our brains and our bodies. While our rudimentary understanding will certainly be refined and modified as we learn more, an excellent description of the current picture is provided in Raphael Cushnir's book, *The One Thing Holding You Back: Unleashing the Power of Emotional Connection.*

It might seem counterintuitive, but an emotional response is a physical response induced by our minds. An emotion causes an involuntary flood of short-lived neurotransmitters and hormones whose purpose is to induce physical changes in our bodies: tightened (or loosened) muscle activation, elevated (or lowered) blood pressure, constriction (or dilation) of our pupils and similar changes that heighten our senses, increase (or decrease) our heart rates, our oxygen consumption, our breathing rate. It is the result of complex neural circuitry. The emotion of happiness, for example, uses an extraordinary array of different regions in the brain, lighting up in complex patterns that differ from person to person.

Often, physical changes arise in our bodies in response to the situation even before we become aware of any conscious thought. More commonly, physical changes occur in response to our thoughts, our mind-created scenarios ruminating over past situations or extrapolating future situations.

We can become aware of the response if we tune-in to our bodies. We feel the heart pound, we feel the blood pressure rise, and we feel the tension in our muscles. If not indicated, as in most situations, the emotional response will be felt, duly noted, and allowed to wash on out. Our bodies and minds then return to the basal state of relaxation and readiness.

That's how it should work. However, all too often, we don't let go of the emotional response cascade. Our thoughts replay the event after the fact, add drama and detail to ramp up the effect, hijack and reroute the release, the letting go back to the basal state.

It doesn't have to be that way. We can take a deep breath and let it go so that our left brain isn't creating a mind-based scenario that is inducing a physical response that is no longer necessary or useful. We can even sigh out the stress.

This is where the MBSR toolkit is very useful. For cultivating and exercising awareness of our "left" brain scenarios and our physical responses to emotional states, then helping to recreate states that are beneficial, be they baseline relaxation states or even consciously arrived at positive states.

Meditation is the practice of becoming aware of our conscious thoughts, of "hearing" the left brain story. Yoga, which comes from a word that means "to yoke", helps to create the awareness of the link, the connection, the yoke between our bodies and our minds. This yoke is often our emotions. Yoga can help us to attune to our emotions (as can other energy work), to feel their embodiment, to become aware of how our bodies relax as our minds relax. Imagery is the practice of cultivating mental states that translate into desired physical states. It is a full-brain (right and left) exercise of conscious induction of emotional-physical responses through imagination.

♀ Key Study: Moffitt Cancer Center

The first randomized, controlled trial of MBSR for breast cancer survivors was published in 2009. Investigators at the Moffitt Cancer Center noted that studies investigating interventions to relieve distress in breast cancer survivors focused primarily on the period around diagnosis and during treatment; few studies looked at relieving symptoms of distress after treatment. The investigators set out to specifically address the major issues of women who are in the first year or so after treatment. Since psychological effects of disruption of life and the resultant fall-out of treatment are predominant problems during this post-treatment period, the investigators sought an intervention that would best address issues of depression, stress, anxiety, and fear as well as potentially improve physical function and overall quality of life. Based on earlier non-randomized studies, they chose MBSR.

The study randomized 84 breast cancer survivors who were within 18 months of having completed their treatment to a six week course of MBSR or a "usual care" control group (3). The course was based on the algorithm developed by Kabat-Zinn. Participants met once weekly, and were also assigned home practice. At the beginning of each week, there was time for open discussion about their experience with MBSR home practice.

A review of the way that the investigators measured outcomes is informative, but rather exhaustive. Participants in the Moffitt study were asked to complete questionnaires both before and at the end of the six week course. Here's what was measured and how (you can try it yourself in the self-assessment at the end of this chapter)

- Fear of recurrence, measured by the 30-item Concerns about Recurrence Scale (CARS) which measures the extent and nature of fears of recurrence.
- Anxiety, measured by the State-Trait Anxiety Inventory, which measures both current and long-term, characteristic anxiety.
- Depression, measured by the Center for Epidemiological Studies Depression Scale.
- Optimism, measured by the Life Orientation Test, which assesses expectancy for positive and negative life outcomes.
- Stress, measured by the Perceived Stress Scale which asks 'how often in the past month has such and such been stressful'.
- Quality of life, measured by the Medical Outcomes Studies Short form General Health Survey. This measures a host of aspects of quality of life, including physical function, role function, pain, general health, vitality, social function, emotional function, and mental health.

- Social support, measured by the Medical Outcomes Social Support Survey, which measures tangible, affectionate, positive social interactions as well as emotional or informational support.
- Spirituality, measured by Likert scores.
- Symptoms of treatment measured by the M.D. Anderson Symptom Inventory.

MBSR proved to have many benefits. Those who were randomized to the mindfulness training course had **less fear, less anxiety, less depression, and better quality of life** than those who did not receive the mindfulness course. In fact, of all the things measured, very few were not affected by mindfulness. For example, social support and spirituality were not affected by mindfulness. Nor was optimism. Mindfulness practice appears to be most effective at improving symptoms of emotional distress that many breast cancer survivors experience in the aftermath of breast cancer diagnosis and treatment.

This ground-breaking trial also demonstrated a few other important points. First, the mindfulness course proved to be quite feasible. The drop-out rate was very low, and the vast majority (85%) attended more than three quarters of the classes. Furthermore, a whopping 97.5% recorded their home practice in a daily diary, meeting the recommended 15-45 minutes per day. The study also showed that those who practiced more had greater benefits in stress reduction, reduced pain, and improved emotional well-being. The body scan exercise and sitting meditation seemed to confer the greatest benefit. It's impressive that 30 minutes per day of sitting quietly and intentionally paying attention to your body can have such far-reaching effects.

❢ *Key Study: British Study*

The second randomized, controlled trial of MBSR in breast cancer patients looked in more detail at breast-cancer related effects, specifically endocrine (hormonal) effects (4). In this British trial of 229 breast cancer survivors who had completed treatment, participants were randomized to an eight week MBSR program ala Kabat-Zinn or to routine followup care. Outcomes were measured by survey questionnaires before the beginning, at the end of the MBSR program, and one month later.

At the beginning of the class, measurements of mood and quality of life were slightly **worse** in the mindfulness training group than in the control group. This was just by chance (randomized studies always look to see whether there are differences between groups at baseline to ensure that the question they are testing is the cause of the later differences). In this case, the groups were not equivalent at the beginning. However, but by the end of the eight week course, the MBSR group had **better** outcomes than the control group despite starting out in a worse place. In other words, not only did the mindfulness training improve outcomes, it improved them enough to make up for being slightly worse off in the beginning. Statistically significant improvements were demonstrated for physical well-being, social well-being, emotional well-being, and functional well-being. Looking more specifically at what was improved the most, the investigators found that depression, anger, fatigue, and confusion were most improved with the mindfulness practice.

The benefits continued even after the course was completed. Significant improvements were still seen three months after completion of the course, particularly in those who practiced more. This larger, confirmatory trial validates the Moffitt study.

The investigators looked further into the physical well-being by asking specifically about breast cancer and hormonal-related symptoms. MBSR improved a diverse range of troublesome treatment effects, such as poor body image, shortness of breath, and pain.

Some of the most problematic side effects of treatment are related to hormonal shifts. Physical symptoms of hot flashes, vaginal dryness, and loss of libido have a significant negative effect on quality of life. Did you know that studies show that up to a quarter of breast cancer survivors don't complete their prescribed course of endocrine therapy? And, that outcomes are worse if they don't? Unfortunately, some women cannot tolerate the treatment and nothing seems to consistently work to mitigate the side effects of endocrine therapy that are so devastating to their quality of life.

The investigators of the British study specifically asked whether MBSR would improve *endocrine-related quality of life*. MBSR had a strong effect on improving symptoms related to treatment-induced menopause, including hot flashes, loss of libido, and vaginal dryness. To date, MBSR appears to be the most effective approach for resolving hot flashes and other negative effects of endocrine therapy.

While this study did not attempt to measure differences in disease outcomes or survival as these were well beyond the scope of the trial, it's not much of a stretch of the imagination to see that if hormonal symptoms can be improved in women taking hormonal therapy like Tamoxifen, Letrozole, or Femara, the ability to tolerate those very effective medications may be improved.

♀ Key Study: Danish Study

Following quickly on the heels of the British study was another randomized controlled clinical trial from Denmark (5). The Danish study recruited participants in a different way, one that may reduce "selection bias" and better represent the average breast cancer survivor. The investigators contacted all of the women who underwent breast cancer surgery during a particular time period from two major hospitals, and invited all to join. Of the 1,200 or so women invited to participate, 336 actually carried out the study. This is helpful information for anyone designing lifestyle programs for breast cancer survivors because it provides a good estimate of the number of breast cancer survivors in the general population who may be interested in complementary alternative health practices.

Despite the longer program (eight weeks instead of the six weeks used in the Moffitt study) and the fact that the women participating had not sought out the trial on their own, completion rates were excellent. This study also added longer-term follow up points to assess outcomes six months and a year after completion of the MBSR program.

The study confirmed and extended the findings of the other studies. Breast cancer survivors who were randomized to the MBSR program had significantly less depression and anxiety than those who were randomized to usual care follow-up. Importantly, the robust improvements persisted through the one year follow up point, long after the program was completed. Such durable results from a time-limited intervention are impressive.

Another important finding from this study was that the benefits of MBSR were greatest in those who had higher levels of anxiety or depression at baseline, those who needed help the most. To pursue this finding further, the investigators looked at different components of depression. Their data suggests that MBSR may help most with depression related to bodily symptoms, such as fatigue or lack of energy. The investigators postulate that this benefit may be a result of the mindfulness training that helps participants to learn to view sensations in new ways, thus reducing their negative associations. This query into potential mechanisms of MBSR is consistent with other studies of MBSR improvements in mental health that indicate that an increased ability to manage mood, decreased rumination, and non-judging or attachment to outcome can result in improved ability to face difficult situations, look at things differently, and feel empowered with a sense of control and ability to take clear action.

♀ Key Study: MBSR vs NEP

These three randomized controlled trials prove that MBSR significantly improves many important components of mental and physical health of breast cancer survivors when compared to usual care, but how does MBSR measure up to other interventions? That was what investigators started asking next.

The Breast Research Initiative for Determining Effective Strategies for Coping with Breast Cancer (BRIDGES) study designed a randomized controlled clinical trial to ask how

MBSR compared to usual care or a nutrition education program (NEP) with regard to improving quality of life and psychosocial outcomes (6). The investigators incorporated a long-term follow up component to the study to look at the duration of effects long after the completion of the programs, at the two year point. They hypothesized that there would be differences in the benefits of MBSR and NEP. Specifically, they hypothesized that quality of life measurements would be higher in those randomized to MBSR than those randomized to NEP, but that social parameters would be improved more with the NEP than the MBSR. They also postulated that active behavioral coping would be higher in both the NEP and MBSR groups compared to the usual care group.

Results showed that MBSR significantly improved quality of life and coping outcomes compared to the nutrition program or to the usual care support. The differences between groups was less at two years than at earlier time points, primarily because at four months and at one year, the usual care group had significantly decreased scores in coping mechanisms over time that rebounded somewhat by two years. This is an important indicator that the time period between treatment and two years after treatment is a time of need for many breast cancer survivors, one that can be well-addressed by MBSR.

Both the NEP and MBSR improved active behavioral and cognitive coping compared to the usual care group. The investigators had hypothesized that NEP would offer greater benefits than MBSR in this particular aspect of coping (feeling empowered to make good lifestyle choices would be expected to do this), but they were surprised to find that MBSR did just as well as NEP.

MBSR trumped NEP in a host of other effects, including improved quality of life (especially factors related to spirituality), reduced depression, hostility, anger, anxiety, unhappiness, and improvement in a sense of control of life, of meaningfulness, and of comprehensibility of life. Some of these psychological aspects remained significantly improved compared to the other two groups at the two year mark, including improvements in anxiety, unhappiness, and a sense of emotional control over the vagaries of life.

The investigators of this study published another report looking more closely at the benefits of MBSR vs NEP on breast cancer patients who had received or were undergoing radiotherapy (7). The hypothesis was that MBSR would also improve psychological effects related to physical symptoms induced by treatment. Indeed, there were additional benefits from MBSR in those receiving radiotherapy, including better quality of life through an enhanced sense of emotional and social/family well-being, greater coping abilities, decreased feelings of helplessness and need for avoidance, and a larger decrease in general psychological distress over time than those some who were not randomly allotted to receive MBSR. Unlike the other effects we've discussed above, these radiation therapy-specific effects were not seen long-term, but primarily during the course of the mindfulness program and radiation treatment.

♀ Key Study: MBSR vs SET

There are other interventions that more specifically address the aspects of psychological and emotional need that MBSR has been shown to improve than nutrition education. How does MBSR measure up to other forms of emotional/psychological support?

Another carefully studied and well-validated form of cancer support is supportive-expressive therapy (SET), a form of group support that focusses on emotional expression. Since both MBSR and SET share a similar group format, size, structure, and contact hours, they would be well-matched for these variables. They differ, however on their content and focus; SET focuses on group support and emotional expression, MBSR on mindfulness, awareness, and acceptance. Would this make a difference?

Carlson and colleagues performed a randomized controlled trial of MBSR vs supportive expressive group therapy (SET), called the MINDSET trial (8). Carlson et al were pioneers of MBSR for breast cancer survivors and published some of the earliest studies that we haven't talked about in light of more recent and more extensive randomized controlled trials. They hypothesized that both interventions would be superior to the control group, but that MBSR would be superior to SET with regard to reducing stress symptoms, whereas SET would be superior to MBSR for improving social support.

What did they find? First, adherence to the eight week program was similar in both the MBSR and SET interventions, with roughly a 30% dropout rate. Second, both SET and MBSR improved overall mood, and did so pretty much to the same extent. Third, as the investigators had hypothesized, MBSR had a significant effect on reducing symptoms of stress, compared with either the SET intervention or the control group. Furthermore, it was a surprisingly large, clinically significant reduction in stress symptoms. This was mirrored by biological changes. The investigators measured cortisol levels, a biological indicator of stress, and found that this stress hormone was reduced in those who received the MBSR intervention.

MBSR also improved overall quality of life compared to usual care. And, finally, surprisingly, MBSR resulted in greater improvements in overall social support compared to SET, the opposite of what the investigators had hypothesized.

Effect size of MBSR

In aggregate, these well-performed randomized controlled clinical trials prove that MBSR programs significantly improve coping mechanisms (including acceptance, mood, and emotional control), facilitate an increased sense of meaning in the face of the adversity of a breast cancer diagnosis, and can improve personal health and recovery factors. Furthermore, these beneficial effects persist long after the program is completed, some for as long as two years. The effects appear to be greatest for those who need help the most. Finally, MBSR is more effective than another proven strategy, expressive therapy. But just how much effect does MBSR have?

Of course, if you are feeling poorly after breast cancer treatment (who isn't?), and MBSR makes you feel better (as it does for most), you may not care too much about quantifying "how effective" the improvements are. But if you are an insurance company debating whether to fund such interventions, or, if as is the case as of this writing, you have to decide whether it's worth paying the often expensive tuition for a MBSR program out of pocket for yourself, you may want to know how it measures up to other options.

One way to measure this is by calculating an "effect size". This is a statistical method of determining the strength of the relationship between two variables across studies. It can translate into a universal term the value the benefits of MBSR compared to usual care across all of the MBSR studies. This universal term, the effect size can then be used to compare effects of different treatments from different studies and different scenarios, such as, say, a specific type of chemotherapy. A generally accepted rule of thumb is that an effect of <0.1 denotes a trivial effect, 0.1-0.3 a small effect, 0.3-0.5 a moderate effect, and 0.5 a large effect.

So, how effective, in this quantitative sense, is MBSR for breast cancer survivors? A meta-analysis performed with all of the available data on MBSR in breast cancer survivors as of November 2011 was performed to answer this question (9). Note that at that time, half of the randomized controlled trials that we've just discussed were not yet completed. Nonetheless, the investigators calculated that the effect size of MBSR on stress was 0.71, on depression was 0.57, and on anxiety 0.733. Note that all of these effects are well into the "large effect" range (over 0.5). Effect sizes of this magnitude are rarely seen with specific treatments.

What can we conclude from these studies? MBSR is an effective intervention to support breast cancer recovery, better than any other readily administered large-scale approach. It significantly improves emotional function and quality of life in breast cancer survivors, particularly for those who are struggling with the "fall-out" of the disruption of their lives and sense of security in the aftermath of breast cancer treatment.

MBSR is an extremely effective intervention, as proven by Level 1 clinical evidence. This is the highest level of proof that exists in the medical world. It is a wonder that MBSR is not incorporated into every breast cancer survivor's recovery program. It is a pity, a loss. It is something that needs to be rectified. You can do that. To all the health care professionals; get out your prescription pads and make the referral to a MBSR Program. Breast cancer survivors, follow through!

Prescription: Part VI

MBSR course x 1

The evidence:

- The Moffitt Cancer Center randomized controlled trial (RCT) demonstrated that a six week MBSR program for breast cancer survivors completing treatment had a high adherence rate and significantly improved symptoms of emotional distress. MBSR reduced fear, anxiety, and depression, while it improved quality of life (3).
- The British RCT demonstrated that an 8-week MBSR program improved physical well-being, social well-being, emotional well-being, and functional well-being. Improvements persisted beyond three months after completion of the program. MBSR improved treatment related effects of poor body image, shortness of breath, and pain. MBSR also significantly improved endocrine-related side effects, a primary endpoint of the trial (4).
- The Danish RCT demonstrated that an eight week MBSR program improved depression and anxiety, particularly in those who were most affected at baseline. Effects persisted beyond one year after completion. MBSR had additional benefits in those who were undergoing or recently had radiotherapy; including improvements in health related and breast cancer related quality of life, as well as measurements of coping (5).
- The BRIGDES trial compared MBSR to a nutrition education program (NEP). MBSR was as effective as NEP at improving measures of coping and empowerment, and was better than NEP (and control) at improving emotional factors (6). Improvements in anxiety, unhappiness, and a sense of emotional control over the

vagaries of life continued beyond two years. There were additional benefits from MBSR in those receiving radiotherapy, including better quality of life through an enhanced sense of emotional and social/family well-being, greater coping abilities, decreased feelings of helplessness and need for avoidance, and a larger decrease in general psychological distress (7).

- In a randomized trial comparing MBSR to Supportive Expressive Therapy (SET), MBSR significantly reduced symptoms of stress. This was accompanied by corresponding changes in cortisol levels. MBSR also improved quality of life, and improved social functioning more than SET (8).

- A meta-analysis of RCTs published as of 2011 calculated the effect size of MBSR. The effect of MBSR on stress was 0.71, on depression was 0.57, and on anxiety 0.733. The effect size of MBSR is large (over 0.5) and clinically relevant for these factors (9).

Alice's MBSR story

Since my mid-thirties, I've been interested in spirituality and our "oneness": connectedness to nature and to each another. I'd like to say that I developed a steadfast practice from those days that has carried me through the good and the bad times of my life. As we all know, life gets in the way and so I find that 20 years later, my spiritual practices are not uniform and not constant. I think of this as a journey and when I say "this", I mean my life, my relationships with my spouse and my children, my breast cancer and treatment and post treatment practices, including mindfulness practices.

I have come to accept and to honor that for me, my "practice" is to seize spiritual moments and I try to do this as frequently as possible. Sometimes, this might involve a morning meditation. Other times, I find myself in a silent meditation as I drive from my home to Charlotte, where I grew up and where I still have family. I have a few like-minded friends who are very encouraging and with whom I practice some types of mindfulness like silent days, Taize service, creating mandalas, or learning Qigong.

One wonderful benefit from having been treated at UNC for breast cancer is that I was able to participate in a program that encouraged not only exercise but also mindfulness. While I'd been interested in mindfulness for some time, it was at UNC that I learned about one of my favorite practices -- HeartMath tools and techniques. You can learn more about HeartMath by going to their website: HeartMath.org. Take the time to listen to the founder's message as it is so encouraging and uplifting. The HeartMath tools I use today are so helpful in lessening and alleviating anxiety, anger and fear, among other things. It's intentionally simple and all based on breathing into your heart to create a state of coherence so that your thoughts are more balanced and internally, you feel more harmonious.

Am I completely proficient, grounded and well-practiced in mindfulness? The answer is no, but I'm accepting that mindfulness work is a moving current that is always available and ready and willing to move me forward as I step in and out of various practices.

Lisa's MBSR story

Like many women, I fell into the trap of multitasking to handle my lengthy professional and personal to-do lists. There is nothing like a breast cancer diagnosis to help you focus on what is truly important on these lists!

Prompted by the New Life Prescription for Healthy Behaviors and with the help of my cognitive behavioral therapist, I have worked to develop mindfulness skills to live in the present and enjoy every day.

I am still a work in progress yet here is what is working for me; I keep a Gratitude Journal. Every day I start my morning by naming three things for which I am grateful. Sometimes big, sometimes small things. A dear cousin found an app I now use to record my gratitude. It's called the Five Minute Journal and I love it! Secondly, meditation. I don't do it every day however I find when I do meditation to start my day I am calmer and more focused. I love the *Oprah and Deepak Chopra 21 Day* series and I even bought the one on *Perfect Health*.

Thirdly, I try to be present. I make a concerted effort to stay present with people and activities. I go to lunch with my girlfriends and put away my phone to engage and enjoy the moment. When I cook, I cook. I enjoy the chopping, the stirring, the smells. When I eat, I eat. I have slowed down to enjoy the taste and texture of my food.

I find I am a happier, calmer person and I think the quality of my relationships has deepened through these practices. The silver lining of a breast cancer diagnosis!

Self-Assessment: Part VI

What is the current status of your emotional health? How much stress are you under? You may be interested in trying out one or more of the questionnaires that investigators used in these studies. It is up to you. Perhaps you will identify areas for which you wish to seek help. If your answers to any of these scales place you in a category of needing help, we strongly urge you to act on this finding and seek professional help. You can still do mindfulness training in addition. Perhaps you will want to pick one or more of these questionnaire surveys as an instrument to track your progress as you develop your mindful attitude toward life.

Health-related quality of life is significantly improved with mindfulness practice. A great way to measure where you stand on this parameter, as well as to follow your progress over time, is to use the medical outcomes studies general health survey. There are several versions of this, but the one that serves our purpose is the 20 question general survey. If you go to the RAND.org website, you can access the form questionnaire by following their link to "surveys". You can fill out the form online, print out your answers, and compare them over time. This is an excellent website to learn more about how the survey instruments are developed, and how they are used. It also gives you further information on how to score. We strongly recommend that you check out the RAND website and their resources.

What is your stress level? The Perceived Stress Scale was used by investigators of at least one of the studies we've discussed. You can try it here, if you like.

Self-Assessment

Perceived Stress Scale

The questions in this scale ask you about your feelings and thoughts **during the last month**. In each case, you will be asked to indicate by circling *how often* you felt or thought a certain way.

Name _____ Date _____

Age _____ Gender (*Circle*): **M   F**   Other _____

0 = Never   1 = Almost Never   2 = Sometimes   3 = Fairly Often   4 = Very Often

1. In the last month, how often have you been upset because of something that happened unexpectedly?	0	1	2	3	4
2. In the last month, how often have you felt that you were unable to control the important things in your life?	0	1	2	3	4
3. In the last month, how often have you felt nervous and "stressed"?	0	1	2	3	4
4. In the last month, how often have you felt confident about your ability to handle your personal problems?	0	1	2	3	4
5. In the last month, how often have you felt that things were going your way?	0	1	2	3	4
6. In the last month, how often have you found that you could not cope with all the things that you had to do?	0	1	2	3	4
7. In the last month, how often have you been able to control irritations in your life?	0	1	2	3	4
8. In the last month, how often have you felt that you were on top of things?	0	1	2	3	4
9. In the last month, how often have you been angered because of things that were outside of your control?	0	1	2	3	4
10. In the last month, how often have you felt difficulties were piling up so high that you could not overcome them?	0	1	2	3	4

Please feel free to use the *Perceived Stress Scale* for your research.

Mind Garden, Inc.
info@mindgarden.com
www.mindgarden.com

References
The PSS Scale is reprinted with permission of the American Sociological Association, from Cohen, S., Kamarck, T., and Mermelstein, R. (1983). A global measure of perceived stress. *Journal of Health and Social Behavior, 24,* 386-396.
Cohen, S. and Williamson, G. Perceived Stress in a Probability Sample of the United States. Spacapan, S. and Oskamp, S. (Eds.) *The Social Psychology of Health.* Newbury Park, CA: Sage, 1988.

MBSR programs also significantly reduce anxiety. A survey instrument used in the clinical trials to measure anxiety was The State-Trait Anxiety Inventory for Adults™ (STAI-AD). You can find that and try it out at mindgarden.com. Go to their index of assessments and search for this one by name. That one is available by purchase only. There are also many interesting assessment tools that you might find useful to assess your present state, as well as your progress as you implement mindfulness practice into your routine.

Call to Action: Part VI

Mindfulness is a better way of living. A MBSR course can set you on the path of making meaningful changes in your life. We all can live our best, happiest, most fulfilling life.

This call to action is to challenge you to take a MBSR course. By now, you are already eating well, exercising regularly, and practicing yoga. In short, you are taking excellent care of your body. Now, let's take care of the rest of you. One MBSR course will set you on the way to a lifelong practice of mindfulness.

Where do you find a MBSR course?

- You can check with your local cancer center (both Duke and UNC have MBSR programs) for courses. These are typically pretty expensive, so they do require a major commitment. You could check to see if there is assistance if you qualify. You can also educate your insurance company about the benefits of MBSR and see whether they will cover your course.
- Advocate for low-cost or insurance-covered courses as a component of breast cancer treatment. Write to cancer centers. Write to the American Cancer Society. Write to your insurance company about expanding coverage. If we all keep trying, it will come.
- Look for upcoming clinical trials. For instance, UNC's Get Real and HEEL program offers exercise and mindfulness programs (heart math). As of this writing, a clinical trial for couples-based mindfulness training is also about to open.

- You don't have to go to an actual class for MBSR based stress reduction program, however. You can purchase Dr. Kabat-Zinn's book, *Full catastrophe living* or tapes, or other similar instructional materials and do the course on your own. There are also web-based courses that teach mindfulness (3).
- Try out a meditation class to go with your yoga. These are offered in most communities, usually inexpensively. They also have the benefit of a group to help support you in your practice. In New Life *after* Cancer's community, for instance, both UNC and Duke offer meditation courses. Balanced Movement Therapy in Carrboro offers a range of yoga and meditation classes. There are many more options.
- Organizations like New Life *after* Cancer also offer programs and retreats that are designed to develop mindfulness practices.

References: Part VI

1) Kabat-Zinn J. An outpatient program in behavioral medicine for chronic pain patients based on the practice of mindfulness meditation: Theoretical considerations and preliminary results. Gen Hosp Psychiatry 1982; 4:33-47.

2) Kabat-Zinn J. Full Catastrophe Living: How to Cope with Stress, Pain and Illness Using Mindfulness Meditation. New York NY, Delacorte, 1990.

3) Legnacher C, Johnson-Mallard V, Post-White J et al. Randomized controlled trial of mindfulness-based stress reduction for survivors of breast cancer. Psycho-Oncology 2009; 18:1261-72

4) Hoffman C, Ersser S, Hopkinson J et al. Effectiveness of mindfulness-based stress reduction in mood, breast- and endocrine-related quality of life, and well-being in Stage 0 to III breast cancer: a randomized, controlled trial. J Clin Oncology 2012; 30:1335-42.

5) Wurtzen H, Oksbjerg Dalton S, Elsass P et al. Mindfulness significantly reduces self-reported levels of anxiety and depression: Results of a randomized controlled trial among 336 Danish women treated for Stage I-III breast cancer. European J of Cancer 2013; 49:1365-73.

6) Henderson V, Clemow L, Massion A et al. The effects of mindfulness-based stress reduction on psychosocial outcomes and quality of life in early-stage breast cancer patients: a randomized trial. Br Cancer Res Treat 2012: 131:99-109.

7) Henderson V, Massion A, Clemow L et al. A Randomized controlled trial of mindfulness-based stress reduction for women with early-stage breast cancer receiving radiotherapy. Integrative Cancer Therapies 2013; 12:404-413.

8) Carlson L, Doll R, Stephen J et al. Randomized controlled trial of mindfulness-based cancer recovery versus supportive expressive group therapy for distressed survivors of breast cancer (MINDSET). J Clin Oncology 2013; 31:3119-26.

9) Zainal N, Booth S, and Huppert F. The efficacy of mindfulness-based stress reduction on mental health of breast cancer patients: a meta-analysis. Psycho-Oncology 22: 1457-65, 2013.

Part VII: Creating an Action Plan for your Life

Did you know that making changes in your life follows a process that can defined by different stages of change?

Did you know that creating an action plan can help you to make and maintain desired lifestyle changes?

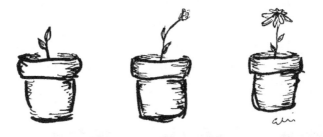

Changing lifestyle behaviors

The data that we have presented is strongly motivating. You can see from medical literature that health behaviors have a very strong impact on breast cancer outcomes, be it risk of recurrence, overall survival, or improved quality-of-life. As you have progressed through this book, we hope that you have taken our recommendations to heart, and initiated healthcare practices that will bring you well-being. You have your prescription for wellness in your hand. It is now up to you.

Of course, these same healthy lifestyle choices can be made by people who have not had cancer and yet many of us are not ready to make the necessary changes that can help us live more optimally. Perhaps the question is not why we choose to ignore healthy lifestyle choices. The question to address is; how can we motivate ourselves into changing our habits, to attain our goals and enjoy the benefits of living healthy?

In our New Life *after* Cancer retreats, we use a method called person centered action planning. It is one way that you can set goals for healthy behavior, and create the structure to back them up. Action planning has been shown to improve the likelihood of successfully completing goals. This section will explore how to get motivated to make changes in our lives, using the action planning process to help us reach our goals.

Stages of change

The Transtheoretical Model of Behavior Change (TTM/Stages of Change) teaches us about the phases that we will likely pass through as we make progress toward changing lifestyle behaviors.

The TTM, commonly known as the *stages of change* is an integrative, biopsychosocial model of chronological phases to guide people through intentional behavior changes (1, 2). The TTM/Stages of Change integrates elements of Bandura's self-efficacy theory, and reflects the level of confidence people have in maintaining their desired behavior change in situations that often trigger relapse into former patterns of behavior (3, 4). It has been shown to be a consistent predictor of the adoption and maintenance of physical activity in adults (5).

There are five stages that people cycle through as they attain their goals. In Prochaska and DiClemente's book, *Changing for Good* (6), they identified the stages of change as *pre-contemplation, contemplation, preparation, action,* and *maintenance*. Each phase of change is distinct and builds upon the other.

The pre-contemplative stage is when an individual doesn't recognize they have a problem, and isn't motivated to make changes that are being recommended by outside sources. If you are reading this far into the book, you are probably well past this stage.

This is followed by the contemplative stage when a person begins thinking about changing a behavior because they believe it may improve their life. We hope that the data you've seen has brought you to this stage and beyond.

The preparation stage is next and uses action planning to define the desired change into steps to implement the change process. Setting goals and breaking them into steps is the exercise within the preparation stage of change, and is integral to the Action Planning process addressed in this chapter. We will cover this in more detail, and guide you through the creation of your own personal action plan.

The next stage is action, and this is when a person practices the new behavior. This stage lasts about three to six months. There are a few pitfalls that can derail this stage. We will offer a few ideas to help to keep you on track during this phase.

The last stage is the maintenance phase. This is when change is fully adopted, we are rarely tempted to return to our old habits, but when we do, we self-correct and return to our previously established healthy habits. Yay!

In later years, a sixth stage of change evolved from the original TTM and it is most frequently identified as the *relapse stage*. A relapse happens when people are tempted on a rare occasion to binge eat, or take a week off from their exercise schedule. *Relapse* can occur even months or years after a person is in the *maintenance* phase, well committed to their healthy lifestyle. However, we are human, and even the most diligent lapse sometimes.

When we relapse, it is important to evaluate, what are our triggers? Has something changed in our life? Have we suffered a loss, or a traumatic life event? By examining what creates the environment that leads to a *relapse*, we can avoid it in the future. Also, there should be an awareness that relapse does not have to result in a long term downward spiral, away from our goal of a healthy life. This is the time to reassess our motivation, call on our friends for support, and start anew.

Stage of Change	Stage Defined	Solutions
Pre-Contemplative	People don't recognize the need to change a behavior. They may listen to people giving them advice on why they should change but they don't make any movement towards changing. Pre-contemplators resist change, they believe a situation is hopeless, and don't believe they can succeed.	Recognize that you may be feeling overwhelmed, de-moralized by past failures. You aren't alone, seek like-minded support Self-examine your ambivalence
Contemplation	People recognize that they have a problem, and they begin to think seriously about resolving it. This phase can last years because people feel "stuck" in this behavior pattern and don't know how to move forward.	Recognize and validate lack of readiness Encourage evaluation of pros and cons of behavior change Identify, encourage and help visualize positive life outcomes as a result of making a change.

Preparation	Change is eminent and will happen within one month People may still feel ambivalent about change Setting defined goals is essential in this phase	Make an Action Plan Identify obstacles Identify supports Identify a timeline for completion of goals Share the plan with others who can support the change process
Action	Practice new behavior for 3 to 6 months	Increase self-efficacy as obstacles arise Rely on support Address feelings of loss, but focus on long term benefits
Maintenance	Continued commitment to new behavior Stage lasts 6 months to 5 years, until individual fully incorporates new change into lifestyle and is rarely tempted to return to former unhealthy lifestyle choices.	Plan and use internal and external support Address relapses to old behaviors Full integration of change into individual's identity

The following table illustrates what our thoughts and actions may be as we consider making healthy life style changes in our life.

Stages of change: Examples of healthy lifestyle changes

Stage	Thought Process	Rationale
Pre-Contemplative	I can continue to live my life as I did in the past, even though I have had breast cancer and even though I notice I don't have the same level of energy.	Cancer happens to millions of people, it doesn't really make a difference if I watch what I eat, exercise and practice mindfulness.
Contemplative	I really don't feel the way I did before I had cancer. I feel exhausted and depressed. Maybe there is something to this notion that healthy living, may improve my quality of life.	I am not sure I can make changes in my life. Perhaps I could make a list of the pros and cons associated with making healthy lifestyle changes. I can meet with other survivors that have made changes to their lives and learn more about how these choices have improved their lives.

Preparation	I can make these changes, because I know I can improve my quality of life for myself and my family.	I will make an Action Plan I will find and participate in a circle of support
Action	I am walking at least three times a week, learning about healthy nutritional choices, and eating well balanced meals.	I have a walking buddy. I have joined a cooking class.
Maintenance	I feel better, I want to continue living my life this way, I really don't want to return to my old way of life.	I have family and friends that participate in activities that reflect healthy lifestyle choices. Sure, once in a while I eat the cheesecake, but the next day, I return to making good nutritional choices.

Pitfalls during maintenance: Beat the blasé factor

Don't let the daily grind wear you down. We all have a much harder time sticking to a health behavior change that we don't like. Exercises we don't enjoy or diets that don't let us eat enough of the foods we crave are much more difficult to sustain. As mentioned above, a goal is that you will feel better when you are doing things that are right for your body. There are many excellent health recommendations that we find are too difficult for all of us. For instance, although a vegetarian diet is healthier and more sustainable for the planet, some of us are not currently ready to give up eating meat. However, we can eat less of it and eat meat that comes from conscientious sources. We believe that it is important to not be too restrictive or too hard on yourself. Take care of yourself by meeting your needs. Give yourself encouragement and praise as you move in the right direction, but don't set yourself up for failure by quitting a healthy habit because you can't do it all the way. Every little bit helps. With time, you will get closer and closer to establishing the healthiest routines.

With that in mind, you will find that most of our recommendations are "to-do", as opposed "to-don't". For instance, we hope that you eat more vegetables. After all, eating more vegetables will probably mean you end up eating less meat. In other cases, we recommend that you avoid something and favor something else. For example, we show you why you might want to avoid omega-6 fatty acid containing meats in favor of omega-3 fatty acid containing meats.

One of the best ways to beat the daily grind aspect of motivation demise is to look at the reasons for continuing. When you review the survival data of women who get more exercise and eat more veggies compared to those who do not, and see the difference it makes in outcomes, you instantly regain motivation. The data and science behind the recommendations is motivating and encouraging. If you know why you should eat your broccoli, it really helps you to choose broccoli over french fries.

The hardest part about change is sustainability and beating the blasé factor. We may have good intentions at the outset, but over time get bored. Perhaps we start to question whether it's really necessary and quietly, we slip back into our old habits.

We are all still learning every day. As we cover the basics, the primary recommendations, we will give variations on the themes. For example, for lymphedema care, we have proven interventions such as manual lymphatic drainage. And now, we have an indication that weight lifting may help. But there are also other options, such as swimming, or dance, or Feldenkrais. We call these derivatives. They are there or you to explore, to spice things up a bit. Pick one or more that you enjoy and use them to augment your basics. New ideas crop up every day. Feel free to try them on for size, to see what you think, but not at the expense of the basics.

Another major way to beat the blasé factor is to enlist friends. Getting a group together to go walking every day not only gives you exercise; it reinforces you to do it. Plus, there's the added bonus of socialization time. That's been proven to benefit mood, energy, well-being, and a host of other positive outcomes. Get together with a few friends to discover new healthy restaurants in your area. Better yet, arrange a potluck lunch or dinner once a month to share your favorite breast cancer healthy recipes. Perhaps you will join us on a New Life *after* Cancer retreat or workshop.

In other words, reinforce your motivation by incorporating others. You can help each other to stick with the program and make some great friends while you do.

Other tools for behavioral change

There are also other behavior change theories and models, validated within the field of dietetics, that offer some explanations for nutrition related behavior change. The research indicates that Motivational Interviewing (MI) has been shown to be a highly effective counseling strategy, especially when paired with cognitive behavioral therapy to support lifestyle changes (7). MI is credited to William R. Miller, Ph.D. who published a paper on his theoretical intervention in 1983 (8). MI helps people who are contemplating a life change access their own natural, internal motivation and capacity for positive action (9). It is an evidence based counseling approach to help people resolve long standing problematic behavior and make changes to these behaviors in a relatively short span of time.

A MI trained therapist asks a series of questions to a client exploring why an individual may be ambivalent towards change. This counseling process eventually helps them identify why they want to change, and supports goal setting that reflect how life will be after the change has occurred. MI has been found to be a highly effective intervention strategy in the areas of substance abuse, and more recently in helping people change other lifestyle habits has been found to be a highly effective intervention strategy in the areas of substance abuse, and more recently in helping people change other lifestyle habits.

Goalsetting, problem solving and social support are also effective methods to making lasting lifestyle changes (7). Other methods to successfully motivate change include self-efficacy, goal setting, and vicarious experiences.

Self-efficacy is defined as the belief that one possesses the stamina to organize and execute a course of action that is necessary to attain a change in their life. It is a key construct in several theories in health psychology, including motivation theory, social cognitive theory and the theory of planned behavior. Techniques that build self-efficacy include vicarious experience, verbal encouragement, feedback on past performance and feedback on comparison to other people's performance. Vicarious experience may be why shows like "The Biggest Loser", are popular on television. Viewers watch each week to see an individual attain a huge weight loss. Watching and sharing in other people's successes may indeed make us more successful in reaching our own goals. Verbal encouragement and feedback on our past performance are also useful motivators of successful weight management programs like Weight Watchers or Over Eaters Anonymous. Feedback on comparison to other people's performance keeps us competitive and adults learn as much from other people's experiences as our own.

Interestingly it is important to note that these strategies are associated with "Action Planning", which reinforces our effort or progress towards our goal and builds self-efficacy (5). Therefore, if we want to change our nutritional and physical health habits, it is imperative that we believe we can do it. If we are pre-contemplative and don't yet believe we can make changes the previously described techniques can build self-efficacy and help achieve our goals. This is encouraging!

Action planning

Action planning is a process that an individual participates in that identifies short and long term goals, prognosticating challenges that may impede progress and identifying sources of inspiration to mitigate challenges on our journey to goal attainment, and lifestyle changes.

Action Planning came from the concept that writing goals down, and periodically revisiting them, increases the likelihood that an individual will attain the goals. Stephen Covey used this concept with the Personal Mission Statement assignment from, *The 7 Habits of Highly Effective People* in which people were asked to write down their life mission statement (10). He encouraged people to carry their mission statement in their wallet or in a purse and to look at it frequently. Covey's book sold 25 million copies and still remains one of the all-time best selling self-help books published to date. The Action Planning process designed for New Life *after* Cancer retreat participants was born out of Covey's personal mission statement activity, and includes more components. Action Plans include short and long term goals, the dates of expected achievement, identifying challenges one may expect to encounter as well as sources of support and inspiration.

Action Planning can be used like a map to follow on our journey to changing our behaviors. It is not sufficient to write a goal, without a detailed step by step plan on how to attain that goal. Setting a specific detailed plan of when, where and how to perform behaviors associated with a goal is the most effective way to bring about a positive change in self-efficacy and healthy lifestyle choices (5). It has been found that setting a specific detailed plan in writing of when, where and how to perform behaviors associated with a change, with directions, and supports to achieve these goals, self-efficacy will develop.

Action planning that is done with careful attention to the detail of a goal, that identifies challenges and support to overcome these barriers, will help people succeed and increase their self-confidence, and thus believe that they can make lifestyle changes. As theories of goal setting suggest, setting specific goals leads to better performance than non-specific goals, for example, "I want to lose 20 pounds" instead of "I want to lose weight". Action Planning defines the goal and the specific details and steps to achieve the goal.

The more confident you are that you can complete a goal for example, eating nutritious meals, drinking less alcohol, exercising regularly and any other goal you may put on your Action Plan the more likely you are to achieve it.

Action planning workshops offered at five New Life *after* Cancer Retreats taught the process to over 50 women. Nineteen New Life *after* Cancer retreat participants participated in a survey that asked them how useful the Action Planning process was in helping them make changes in their life. The results indicated that 94% of the participants agreed that Action Planning was a useful process in helping them set and meet their goals and 93% of them continued to use Action Planning to help them identify and achieve new goals.

Our action plan stories

"Each year that I participated (in New Life *after* Cancer retreats) I accomplished at least two of my Action planning goals. A few are that I got in shape; I incorporated yoga and mindfulness activities into my daily life to reduce stress. I completed some advanced education that I had thought about for years, and I sought out a new position to expand on my previous career experience."

"I keep a gratefulness journal now and I am focusing on the positives in my life. I am carving time out for myself each day, without feeling guilty. I am doing exercise and yoga to regain strength and reduce stress."

"I am doing yoga at least two times per month and doing meditation. I have also downsized the amount of clutter in my home and am more able to enjoy it as a result."

"I am travelling more to exotic places and cultures, as a result of one of my action planning goals. In my personal life I continue to reach out to my son, who is estranged from me."

"I made a goal to take some time each week just for me, and I do it!"

"I carve out more time in my life **for me**. I am finding more balance among my many responsibilities as a mother, a wife and a business owner. I have established routines that support a healthier lifestyle including better nutrition."

"I set a number of goals and achieved them all. One was to get a dog and start walking and enjoying exercise again. Another was to lose some of the weight I gained during cancer. I also identified a new career goal, and I am giving my first ever yoga retreat at Emerald Isle this weekend. Another was to prioritize my time better and in a way that makes my life more fulfilling. I completed yoga instruction training, with a master and went to India this year. It's very satisfying to look back and see the goals I set, and what has been accomplished, and for these reasons, I would like to go on another New Life *after* Cancer retreat."

"I was motivated to make a huge career change, inspired by other women on the cruise. I applied to and was accepted to the UNC Law School, where I am now in my final year. It has been a tremendously positive experience. I hope to focus on some aspect of Health Law."

"I have been able to let go of negative influences, and reduced stress with an exercise schedule and travel."

"As a result of the action planning process I participate in regular exercise and a slow but steady weight loss."

"I retired! I also lost a considerable amount of weight and participate in yoga weekly."

"I set my action planning goal on eventual retirement, and I am progressing towards that end. I am also able to enjoy my grandbaby and family more, which makes me happy."

"I quit my full time job which was very stressful and I took on part time employment at a place that I enjoy working. I also find new ways to "do" and "view" in activities that I enjoyed before I had breast cancer. I can modify the activity or participate differently or at my own pace, so I enjoy it without exhausting myself. I also am back to exercising, and I am feeling better about that."

Call to Action: Part VII

People have an infinite number of reasons why they should change a life style habit, yet their goals are often similar: to increase the length and quality of their life. Even when confronted with a life threatening illness, it can be difficult to get motivated to give up an unhealthy lifestyle. Yet, a small voice deep within us may urge us to press on, to find the desire, courage, knowledge and strength to persevere and to set new goals and finally meet them. Our final call to action is to create your own action plan.

Let's walk through the process, as you create your own action plan. The Action Plan Form is included here and may be copied as needed. An example of a completed Action Plan has also been included in this publication.

The Action Planning process begins by identifying two long term goals and two short term goals. Long term goals take more than six months to complete and short term goals can be achieved in less than six months.

Next, ask yourself these questions provided to guide you in the Action Planning process. You will want to answer the questions first, and then try designing your own Action Plan:

- What are your personal strengths, gifts or talents?
- Who are the people that you trust to help you attain your goals?
- What are the characteristics of the people you trust?
- Who may be a support in helping you achieve your action plan that you have not previously considered?
- What activities in your life have you considered trying but have not yet done?

- Why? What are barriers or challenges that have held you back?
- Identify creative strategies that you can use to help you break down those barriers or challenges?
- Identify two healthy lifestyle goals you can accomplish in less than 60 days.
- Identify two healthy lifestyle goals you want to accomplish in six months to a year.
- How will you reward yourself when you accomplish your goals?
- Complete the Action Planning form, and review it frequently to check in on your progress. Remember to CELEBRATE your successes!

Goal	Action Steps What will be done?	Your strengths	Your circle of support or resources	Potential Barriers	Start Date	Goal Date
Short Term Goal I want to eat healthy food daily and get rid of junk food from my diet.	Read New Life *after* Cancer book Attend a class or workshop Stop buying fast food Purchase healthy food	I am motivated I want to have more energy to enjoy life.	My partner My best friend	Hectic schedules Not having time to cook Family likes fast food	Oct 2016	Jan 2017
Long Term Goal I want to lose 25 pounds.	Join Weight Watchers Attend weight manage-ment program weekly Weigh myself every other day	Want to buy fun new clothes Want to have energy to enjoy life Have lost weight success-fully before	My partner My support group and facilitator of the group My neighbor	Temptation to over eat when stressed Holidays or Celebra-tions Procrastin-ation and missing support group meetings	Oct 2016	April 2017

Goal	Action Steps What will be done?	Your strengths	Your circle of support or resources	Potential Barriers	Start Date	Goal Date

Concluding remarks

We have provided information about why we are ambivalent to change, what changes ambivalence to a desire to change and finally what catapults us into action. Evidence based theories, such as the Transtheoretical Model of Behavior Change, and its Stages of Change were described to help us understand the process people go through as they move from an attitude of not caring about changing to making lifestyle changes that become a habit in their daily routine. We have also looked at behavioral health interventions that can be effective at helping us make changes especially when we don't know how, or we don't care enough about making the change. Motivational Interviewing, is a counseling technique practiced by therapists trained in the utilization of a series of questions that help people recognize a need to change and helps set a plan of action in place to model positive change. Motivational Interviewing can be effective in as few as three to five sessions with a skilled therapist. Nutritional and dietetic journal articles, including those that provided a Meta analyses identified behaviors, beliefs and activities that can make people more successful when trying to achieve a goal. Lastly, Action Planning was discussed as a written plan of short and long term goals to keep people on task as they achieve the ultimate goal, an improved quality of life made possible with healthy lifestyle changes.

- TTM/Stages of Change identify five stages people go through when they make changes in their life. People can be stuck in the pre-contemplative and contemplative stages for long periods of time, even years. Counselling with a therapist trained in Motivational Interviewing can help people move from the pre-contemplative (I don't need to change) and contemplative (I may need to change) stages to actually preparing, planning, and finally making the desired change.

- Self-efficacy, or the belief that one can make a change is an important personal characteristic to possess, and research indicates that people with higher levels of self-efficacy make more successful healthy life style changes. For example, if you believe you can lose 10 pounds you are more likely to lose the weight, than someone that does not believe they have the will power to lose the weight.

- If low self-efficacy is a problem there are ways to increase personal confidence. These techniques include watching other people be successful, verbal encouragement, feedback on how a person is doing as they try to meet a goal, and feedback on how a person is doing compared to their peers who are also trying to achieve a similar goal. Using a buddy or friend who is trying to achieve a similar goal can help you both be more successful. As you try to make changes using any or some of these approaches may help you build your confidence and belief that you can achieve your goals.

- Action Planning can help you identify your goals, by writing them down, and providing deadlines to help you move from the planning to the action stage. Action Planning makes us move past ambivalence about change, because it is a written document with concrete steps to follow to achieve our lifestyle changes. Action Planning includes identifying barriers we may encounter as we try to make changes and the people who can be our source of support to push past the challenges.

- Copy the Action Plan in this book, and review the Action Planning questions provided to help you develop your own unique plan. When you have achieved a goal celebrate your progress, reward yourself for a job well done! Recognizing your progress is important not only for you but for someone else, because your success may motivate them to try some new healthy lifestyle changes of their own.

References: Part VII

1) Prochaska, J.O., Diclemente, C.C. &Norcross, J.C. (1992). In search of how people change: applications to the addictive. *American Psychologist, 47*, 1102-1114. PMID: 1329589

2) Noar, S.M., Benac, C.N., & Harris, M.S. (2007). Does tailoring matter? Meta-analytic review of tailored print health behavior change interventions. *Psychological Bulletin, 4*, 673-693. abstract.

3) Bandura, A. (1977). Self-efficacy: toward a unifying theory of behavioral change. *Psychological Review, 84*(2), 191-215. Retrieved from http://psycnet.org

4) Bandura, A. (1982). Self-efficacy mechanism in human agency. *American Psychologist, 37*(2), 122-147. Retrieved from http://psycnet.org

5) Williams, S.L. & French, D.P. (2011). What are the most effective intervention techniques for changing physical activity self-efficacy and physical activity behavior—and are they the same. *Health Education Research, 26*(2), 308-322. Retrieved from http://oxfordjournals.org

6) Prochaska, J.O., Norcross, J.C., & Diclemente, C.C. (1994). *Changing for good.* New York: Avon Books
behaviors. *American Psychologist, 47*, 1102-1114. PMID: 1329589

7) Spahn, J.M., Reeves, R.S., Keim, K.S., Laquatra, I., Kellogg, M., Jortberg, B., & Clark, N.A. (2010). State of the evidence regarding behavior change theories and strategies in nutrition counseling to facilitate health and food behavior change. *Journal of the American Dietetic Association, 110*(6), 879-891. Retrieved from http://sciencedirect.com

8) Miller, W.R. & Rollnick, S. (2013). *Motivational interviewing: helping people change (application of motivational interviewing)* (3rd ed). New York, NY: The Guilford Press.

9) Zuckoff, A. & Gorscak, B. (2015). Finding your way to change: How the power of motivational interviewing can reveal what you want and help you get there. New York, London: The Guilford Press

10) Covey, S.R. (1989). *The seven habits of highly effective people: restoring the character ethic.* New York, NY: Simon and Schuster.

Afterward

There are plenty of additional subjects that we could raise. In our New Life *after* Cancer cooking workshops, we have great fun as we delve more into the science behind specific foods that have been shown in laboratory studies to inhibit or kill breast cancer cells (yes, we cook and discuss science). We could discuss supplements, such as vitamin D, and the evidence that this might play a role in breast cancer. We could raise the issue of soy products and other phytoestrogens on hormonal interactions the breast-cancer survivors. We could describe other than mindful movement practices besides yoga, such as qigong, tai chi, or Feldenkrais, practices that we introduce in New Life *after* Cancers movement workshops. We could discuss the value of gratitude practice in improving happiness. These and more are all worthy subjects for discussion and research, and with your support, can be the topics of future workshops and books.

There is much still to learn, but this book is the foundation. The subjects that we have covered are all extremely well validated in medical literature. They are "must do's" for the breast cancer survivor who wants to improve her outcomes. We entreat every healthcare provider to hand to every breast cancer survivor a prescription for wellness.

We hope that every breast cancer survivor who reads this book has been motivated by the knowledge. The interventions that we have studied all build upon each other, and if you have been carrying out the recommended practices, we are confident that you are already seeing a big improvement. Keep up the good work!

It takes a village. There is a saying, "It takes a village to raise a child". We are hardwired since ancient times to work together. Our workshops and retreats show us that breast-cancer survivors thrive when they work together toward health and wellness. It is very important to supplement your practices with support from friends, from family, from community. Our final call to action is to urge you to create for yourself a community of support for your healthy lifestyle.

It takes a village to develop and continue New Life *after* Cancer as well. We are grateful for the hard work and financial support of a handful of people who have me this project possible. We are also grateful to UNC/Lineberger and the V Foundation for providing the startup funds for New Life *after* Cancer.

If this book has helped you, buy another one and give it to a friend. Or buy several copies and put them in your cancer center or your clinic waiting room. Or donate to New Life *after* Cancer so that we can provide the book to those who ask for it. If you would like to help us to produce video recordings of the companion lectures from the New Life *after* Cancer workshops and retreats that are the foundation of this book, please consider making a tax-deductible donation to New Life *after* Cancer. All proceeds from the purchase of this book and donations go directly toward New Life *after* Cancer's educational programs. Please support and grow your community.

Made in the USA
Las Vegas, NV
02 December 2021

35830638R00162